Essence of
TRADITIONAL
CHINESE MEDICINE

中医

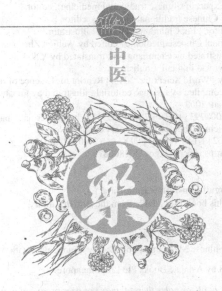

Compiled by Asiapac Editorial

Editorial Consultants
Dr. Zhu Wenjun
Singapore College of Traditional Chinese Medicine, Singapore

Dr. Lin Yuan
Dr. Cheng Sim Kim

Illustrated by
Fu Chunjiang

Translated by
Y N Han

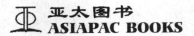
亚太图书
ASIAPAC BOOKS

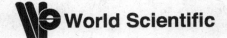
World Scientific

Published and distributed by

World Scientific Publishing Co. Pte. Ltd.
5 Toh Tuck Link, Singapore 596224
USA office: 27 Warren Street, Suite 401-402, Hackensack, NJ 07601
UK office: 57 Shelton Street, Covent Garden, London WC2H 9HE

Library of Congress Cataloging-in-Publication Data
Names: Zhu, Wenjun (Expert in Chinese traditional medicine), editor. |
    Lin, Yuan (Expert in Chinese traditional medicine), editor. |
    Cheng, Sim Kim, editor. | Fu, Chunjiang, 1974–   illustrator.
Title: Essence of traditional Chinese medicine / edited by Wenjun Zhu, Yuan Lin,
    Sim Kim Cheng ; illustrated by Chunjiang Fu ; translated by Y.N. Han.
Other titles: Zhonghua yi yao jing cui. English
Description: New Jersey : World Scientific, 2018. | Reprint of: Essence of traditional
    Chinese medicine / compiled by Asiapac editorial ; illustrated by Fu Chunjiang ;
    translated by Y.N. Han. 2003.
Identifiers: LCCN 2018008793 | ISBN 9789813239180 (hardcover : alk. paper)
Subjects: | MESH: Medicine, Chinese Traditional | Graphic Novels
Classification: LCC R602 | NLM WB 17 | DDC 615.8/80951--dc23
LC record available at https://lccn.loc.gov/2018008793

British Library Cataloguing-in-Publication Data
A catalogue record for this book is available from the British Library.

Essence of Traditional Chinese Medicine. Published by arrangement with Asiapac Books Pte Ltd.

Copyright © 2003, 2018 by Asiapac Books Pte Ltd, Singapore

For any available supplementary material, please visit
http://www.worldscientific.com/worldscibooks/10.1142/10962#t=suppl

Typeset by Stallion Press
Email: enquiries@stallionpress.com

Printed in Singapore

Other Related Titles from World Scientific

Essential Chinese Medicine
(A 4-Volume Set)
Volume 1: Restoring Balance
Volume 2: Health Tonics
Volume 3: Improving Blood Circulation
Volume 4: Relieving Wind
by Bao Chun Zhang and Yu Ting Chen
ISBN: 978-981-3239-06-7 (Vol. 1)
ISBN: 978-981-3239-09-8 (Vol. 2)
ISBN: 978-981-3239-12-8 (Vol. 3)
ISBN: 978-981-3239-15-9 (Vol. 4)

Anecdotes of Traditional Chinese Medicine
by Lifang Qu
edited by Mary Garvey
ISBN: 978-1-938134-99-9
ISBN: 978-1-945552-02-1 (pbk)

Tu Youyou's Journey in the Search for Artemisinin
by Wenhu Zhang, Yiran Shao, Dan Li and Manyuan Wang
translated by Junxian Yu
ISBN: 978-981-3207-63-9
ISBN: 978-981-3207-64-6 (pbk)

Cancer Management with Chinese Medicine: Prevention and
Complementary Treatments
Revised Edition
by Rencun Yu and Hong Hai
ISBN: 978-981-3203-88-4
ISBN: 978-981-3231-85-6 (pbk)

Ginseng and Ginseng Products 101: What are You Buying?
by Hwee Ling Koh, Hai Ning Wee and Chay Hoon Tan
ISBN: 978-981-4667-30-2
ISBN: 978-981-4667-31-9 (pbk)

Publisher's Note

Traditional Chinese medicine has a long history, and it is known throughout the world for its unique methods of diagnosis and treatment. Some of the fundamental concepts of traditional Chinese medicine are already part of our ingrained habits. During the hot summer months, we drink herbal tea to cool down; when the weather turns cold, we consume tonics; when we feel flushed and dry in the mouth, we consume cooling foods; but when our lips and nails are pale, it is a sign of anaemia, so we consume foods that will replenish the blood....

It is our hope to make the world of traditional Chinese medicine accessible to everyone. The book explains the fundamental theories behind traditional Chinese medicine with the help of easy-to-understand diagrams, covers the methods of diagnosis and treatment, and introduces famous historical physicians who influenced the development of traditional Chinese medicine.

This book is the product of a collaborative effort on the part of the Asiapac editorial team to research and compile materials in consultation with authorities on traditional Chinese medicine. Special thanks go to Mr Zhu Wenjun, Dr Lin Yuan and Dr Cheng Sim Kim for their invaluable contributions.

We also wish to thank Mr Fu Chunjiang for his vibrant illustrations, Ms Y N Han for the translation and Mr Zhu Wenjun for writing the foreword. At the same time, we would like to thank Mr Huang Ruide for his assistance, Ms Wong Wan Ling for her editorial support and Ms Wu Li Bin for providing information on Chinese medical bodies in Singapore. Finally, we wish to thank the production team for their hard work that has made this publication possible.

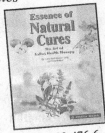
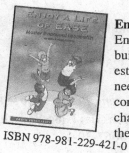

Foreword

Traditional Chinese medicine is a treasure of the Chinese civilization and an unique aspect of Chinese science and technology, with a history going back thousands of years. The tireless efforts of our forefathers have helped it develop into a unique branch of medicine. Though it originated in China, traditional Chinese medicine is an asset to the human race. To benefit the greatest number of people, it has to go global.

It came to Singapore with the early Chinese immigrants. But that was only a spontaneous situation. With the development of Chinese medicine and government emphasis on the training and development of traditional Chinese medicine in the eighties and nineties, interest and confidence in traditional Chinese medicine increased. While some opted for overseas training, others stayed home to study this branch of medicine. It is with the purpose of acquainting Singaporeans with Chinese medicine that this book has been published. At the same time, it is also in keeping with the current trend of going 'back to nature'.

Essence of Traditional Chinese Medicine provides a comprehensive and in-depth coverage of traditional Chinese medicine. Topics ranging from theories, practical experience and traditional material to modern technology offer a good foundation for understanding traditional Chinese medicine. Diagrams and illustrations enhance understanding of the text. The practical aspect is made relevant and applicable; stories of famous physicians are put across in a lively manner. All these make this book an easy and informative read.

This book is not only for beginners or those who want a general guide to traditional Chinese medicine. It is also a good companion to families, with simple and effective tips to preserve health, underlining the importance of a healthy lifestyle, prevention of premature ageing and longevity.

Zhu Wenjun
Dean
TCM College (S) Pte Ltd
May 2003

Zhu Wenjun holds a Masters degree from China Pharmaceutical University and taught at Nanjing University of Traditional Chinese Medicine.

Contents

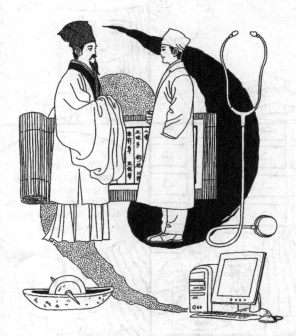

Prologue

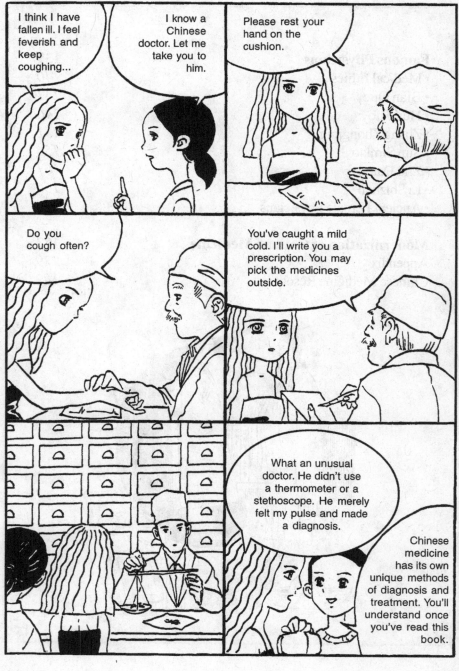

THE CONCEPT AND THEORY BEHIND CHINESE MEDICINE

The art of Chinese medicine has a history that goes back a few thousand years. It integrates the concepts of yin and yang, five elements, and the union of man and nature in Chinese philosophy into a unique theory and system that stands as one of a kind in the medical world. Its outstanding therapeutic efficacy has also gained widespread recognition.

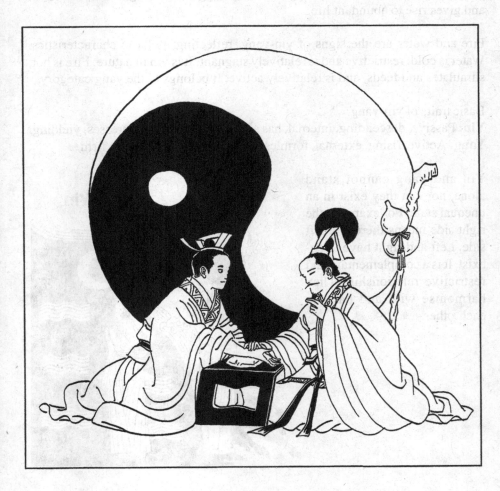

Yin and Yang

Everything in creation is categorised into yin (vital essence) and yang (vital energy). For example, in the celestial system, the moon is yin while the sun is yang. In the human system, females are yin while males are yang. The interaction of yin and yang induces changes and causes life on earth to proliferate. Yin and yang complement each other. Together, they trigger off changes in the universe and gives rise to abundant life.

Fire and water are the signs of yin-yang, reflecting its basic characteristics. Water is cold, restrictive and is relatively stagnant. It is yin in nature. Fire is hot, stimulates and feeds, and is relatively active. It belongs to the yang category.

Basic traits of yin-yang:
Yin: Passive, descending, internal, has a form, cold, dark, suppresses, yielding.
Yang: Active, rising, external, formless, warm, bright, stimulates, firm.

Yin and yang cannot stand alone, nor can they exist in an unequal state. For example, the right side means there is a left side. Left and right have to co-exist. It is a complementary and restrictive relationship. They harmonise with and balance each other.

Yang　　　　**Yin**

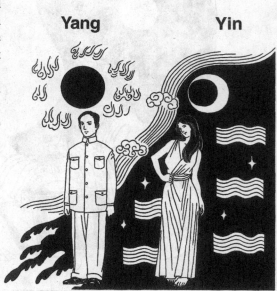

Application in Chinese medicine

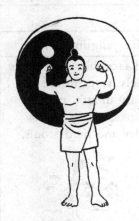 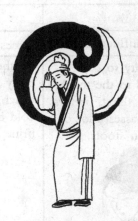 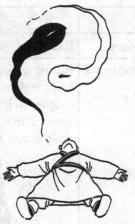

When a person's yin and yang are in balance, there is good health.

When the yin and yang are not in balance, there is ill health.

When yin and yang leave the body, death comes.

The makeup of the human body is also categorized into yin and yang:

The upper body is yang; the lower body is yin.

The exterior is yang; the interior is yin.

The back is yang; the chest and abdomen are yin.

The heart, liver, spleen, lungs and kidneys are yang; the stomach, gallbladder, intestines and bladder are yin.

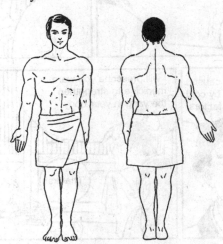

Ailments may be classified as yin and yang as well:

	Yin Syndrome	Yang Syndrome
Causes	Excessive yin influences.	Excessive yang influences.
Symptoms	Pallor, sensitivity to cold, body feels cold to the touch, fatigue, lack of thirst, prefers warm drinks, passes a lot of clear urine, thin stools.	Flushed face, bloodshot eyes, body feels warm to the touch, dry mouth, prefers cold drinks, passes yellow urine, dry and hard stools.

A case study

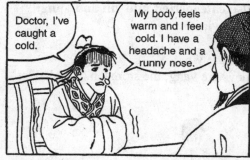

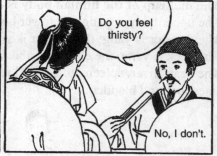

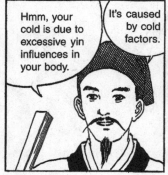

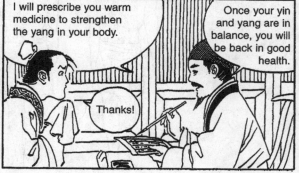

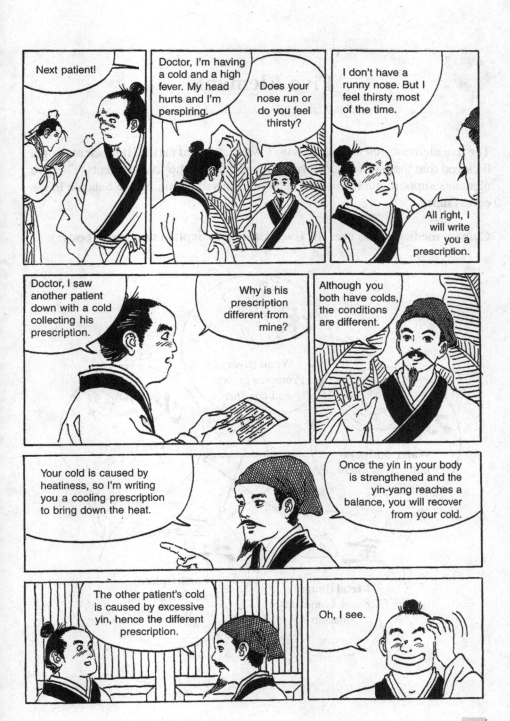

Five Elements

The five elements refer to metal, wood, water, fire and earth. The ancient people believed that the physical universe was made up of the five elements. The five elements support and oppose one another, thus maintaining the balance in the eco-system.

Chinese medicine also uses the five elements to explain the human body:

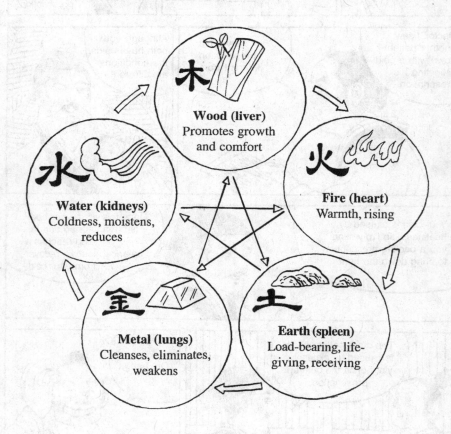

木
Wood (liver)
Promotes growth and comfort

火
Fire (heart)
Warmth, rising

水
Water (kidneys)
Coldness, moistens, reduces

金
Metal (lungs)
Cleanses, eliminates, weakens

土
Earth (spleen)
Load-bearing, life-giving, receiving

The constructive and inhibitive relationships among the Five *Zang*, or vital organs.

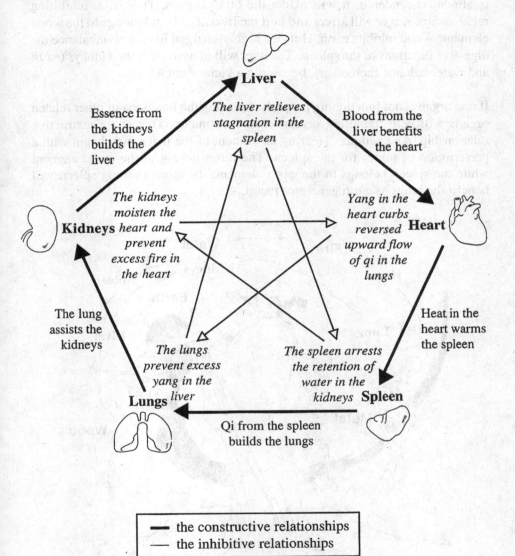

Liver

Essence from the kidneys builds the liver

The liver relieves stagnation in the spleen

Blood from the liver benefits the heart

The kidneys moisten the Kidneys *heart and prevent excess fire in the heart*

Yang in the heart curbs reversed upward flow of qi in the lungs Heart

The lung assists the kidneys

The lungs prevent excess yang in the Lungs *liver*

The spleen arrests the retention of water in the kidneys Spleen

Heat in the heart warms the spleen

Qi from the spleen builds the lungs

── the constructive relationships
── the inhibitive relationships

The Five *Zang* support and inhibit one another

If one organ is infected or suffers internal injuries, ailments will arise. If no treatment is rendered, it will affect the other organs. This is an inhibiting relationship: Anger will affect and hurt the liver. The liver belongs to the wood element. Wood inhibits earth. Hence a highly-charged liver will unbalance the digestive functions of the spleen. The liver will in turn affect the kidneys (earth and water balance each other), becoming a vicious circle.

If one organ is not functioning properly, boosting the functions of other related organs will help the ailing organ resume normalcy. This is a constructive relationship. An example: Treating an ailment of the lungs may begin with a prescription of tonics for the spleen. The lungs belong to the metal element while the spleen belongs to the earth element; therefore a strong spleen will benefit the lungs as earth generates metal.

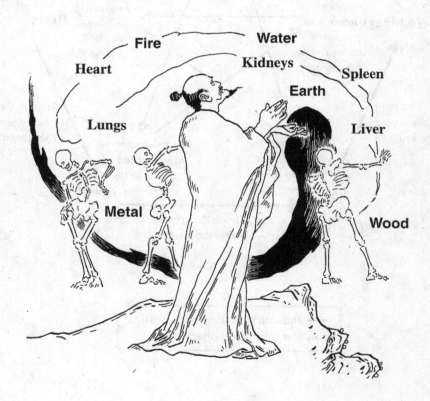

Categorisation of Objects and Phenomena
According to the Five Elements

Five Elements					
	Wood	**Fire**	**Earth**	**Metal**	**Water**
Nature					
Seasons	Spring	Summer	Late Summer	Autumn	Winter
Directions	East	South	Center	West	North
Climate	Wind	Summer Humidity	Dampness	Dryness	Coldness
Changes	Germinate	Grow	Transform	Harvest	Store
Color	Green	Red	Yellow	White	Black
Flavors	Sour	Bitter	Sweet	Pungent	Salty
Tones	Jiao	Zheng	Gong	Shang	Yu
Human Body					
Five Senses	Eye	Tongue	Mouth	Nose	Ear
Zang Fu	Liver	Heart	Spleen	Lung	Kidney
	Gall Bladder	Small Intestine	Stomach	Large Intestine	Urinary Bladder
Tissue	Tendon	Vessel	Muscle	Skin, Hair	Bone
Emotions	Anger	Joy	Thinking	Melancholy	Fear
Sound	Shout	Laugh	Sing	Cry	Mourn

The Premise of Chinese Medicine

The human body as a unified system

Chinese medicine sees the human body as the sum of various parts that are linked to one another. Every organ, main and collateral channel, qi and blood flow does not function independently. Rather, they are interdependent. Hence, when there is a change to any one part, the other parts will be affected as well. In the diagnosis of ailments, the body is treated as a whole. External observation will assist in the diagnosis of internal ailments. Any treatment that follows should consider the interrelationships before it is recommended.

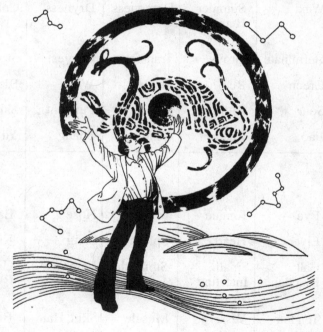

The close relationship between man and environment

Natural factors like changes in the climate, time of the day, geographical locations affect human biological activities, bodily changes as well as the diagnosis and treatment of ailments to a certain extent. Nature is therefore regarded as part of the human makeup. They are interlinked.

Eight Principal Syndromes

In traditional Chinese medicine, illnesses can be grouped into 'Eight Principal Syndromes': Yin-Yang, Exterior-Interior, Cold-Heat and Deficiency-Excess.

Yin-Yang:
The primary syndrome among the Eight Principal Syndromes. Exterior, Heat and Excess belong under Yang; Interior, Cold and Deficiency belong to Yin. (Yin-Yang will be explained further in the following pages).

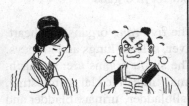

Exterior-Interior:
Some illnesses move from the surface into the interior. An illness at the exterior stage is trifling and is easily treated.
Once an illness invades the interior, it means the illness has become serious.

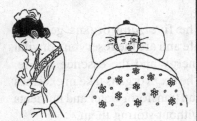

Cold-Heat:
The symptoms of cold are cold limbs, clear urine and pallor. The syndromes of heat include a flushed face, warm body, high irritability and constipation.

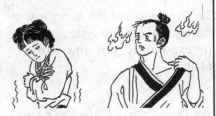

Deficiency-Excess:
Deficiency is marked by deficiency in qi and blood, a weak constitution, loss of weight, giddy spells etc. Excess is marked by symptoms such as rapid breathing, irritability and constipation.

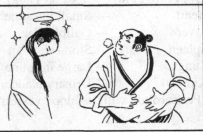

The Viscera (the Internal Organs — Five *Zang* and Six *Fu*)

The viscera are the internal organs in a human body. They are classified into five *zang* organs and six *fu* organs:

The five *zang* organs are: heart, liver, spleen, lungs and kidneys. The six *fu* organs are: stomach, small intestine, large intestine, gallbladder, urinary bladder and Triple Energiser.

The five *zang* organs generate life and are the reservoirs of vital energy and the essence of life. The six *fu* organs take in excesses and transform water and nutrients without storing them.

The five *zang* and six *fu* organs (the viscera) are one system with corresponding yin and yang balances.

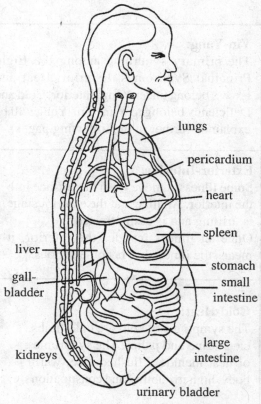

An ancient anatomical diagram showing the various organs of the body. It has some differences from modern diagrams.

Five *Zang* (Yin) — Six *Fu* (Yang)
Heart — Small intestine
Liver — Gallbladder
Spleen — Stomach
Lungs — Large intestine
Kidneys — Urinary bladder
*Pericardium with its blood vessels — Triple Energiser

Pericardium with its blood vessels: also known as shan zhong, *it refers to the membrane (pericardium) surrounding the heart. It serves to protect the heart.*

Controls activity and function of viscera.

Circulates blood and qi in the body, transporting nutrients to other parts of the body.

Perspiration is known as the fluid of the heart.

When the heart functions well and there is ample blood and fluids, one has rosy cheeks; when there is deficiency of blood and fluids, the face turns pale.

Heart

Stores and regulates blood volume.

Regulates the flow of qi, which affects the emotions.

The soul and the spirit have the blood as their foundation. As the liver stores blood, it also stores the soul.

Deficiency of yin and blood in the liver or excess of yang in the liver will cause irritability in a person.

Sufficient blood in the liver will show in strong and pink nails; insufficient blood in the liver will show in thin, soft and pale nails.

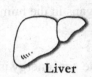

Liver

Controls digestion and transport: Helps digest and absorb nutrients to be distributed through the body. Also transports bodily fluids and maintains fluid balance.

Regulates the flow of blood in the blood vessels:

Helps nourish the limbs and muscles. A healthy spleen will mean strong limbs and muscles. Controls the flow of blood in the arteries and veins. Prevents bleeding.

Ample qi and blood will show in red and lustrous lips; deficiency of blood in the spleen will result in pale lips.

Spleen

In charge of qi. Take in fresh air and expel carbon dioxide and other gases to maintain metabolism.

Regulate the movement of fluids and qi in the body; a fall directs qi downwards to the kidneys and urinary bladder to maintain the normal flow and expulsion of bodily fluids.

All blood in the body flows through the lungs to exchange fresh and stale air before travelling to other parts of the body.

Healthy skin reflects good lung function and is more resistant to pathogens.

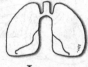

Lungs

Store the essence of the five *zang* and six *fu* organs. It is the basis of life that keeps life activity going.

Regulate water metabolism and control the distribution and expulsion of water and maintain water metabolism within the body.

Thick and glossy hair reflect young and healthy kidneys, while hair loss reflects weak and old kidneys.

Kidneys

Qi (Vital Energy), Blood and Bodily Fluids

Qi, blood and bodily fluids are the primary components that make up and sustain the human body. They are the basis on which the normal function of all the organs in the human body depend.

Qi

The vital energy is the basic element of life in a human body. Our vital energy is constantly circulating, rising, falling, getting expelled and being absorbed. We call these movements the 'qi mechanism'. The 'qi mechanism' refers to the increase, decrease and movement of qi, ie the physiological action of qi. A balanced qi mechanism maintains normal physiological activities. When the qi is out of balance, as when blockage in the qi flow results in a steep increase in the levels of qi and pent-up qi, it will lead to illnesses.

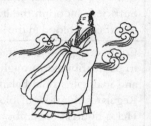

Blood and Bodily Fluids

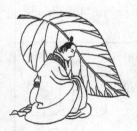

The circulation of blood in the vessels serves to provide nutrients and moisture to the organs. This maintains normal physiological activities. A glowing complexion, glossy hair and firm muscles indicate a healthy blood circulation. The reverse will be manifested in symptoms such as giddy spells, a sallow complexion, dry hair, dry skin, forgetfulness and unconsciousness.

The bodily fluids comprise fluids from the various organs and normal bodily secretions. These fluids keep the internal organs moist and may also transform into blood. Hence, an excessive expenditure of bodily fluids will lead to weak qi and blood circulation. Certain conditions like vomiting, diarrhoea and profuse perspiration will also lead to the depletion of bodily fluids. At the same time, shortness of qi, a pallid complexion and heartburn may manifest.

Main and Collateral Channels, Acupuncture Points

The main and collateral channels transport qi and blood, connects the organs, limbs and joints and are the interface between the exterior and the interior. The main and collateral channels have their designated order and related organs. They are able to reflect any ailment associated with the relevant organs.

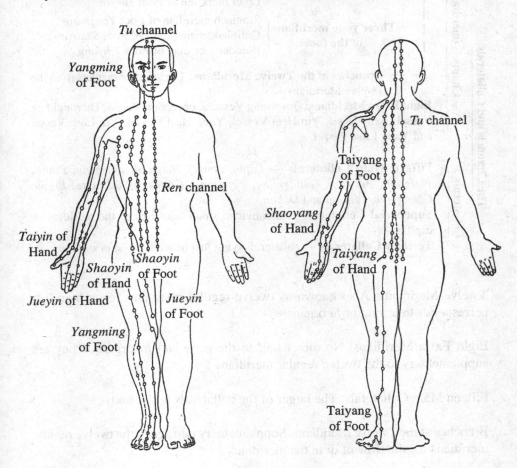

A Summary of the Channels and Collaterals

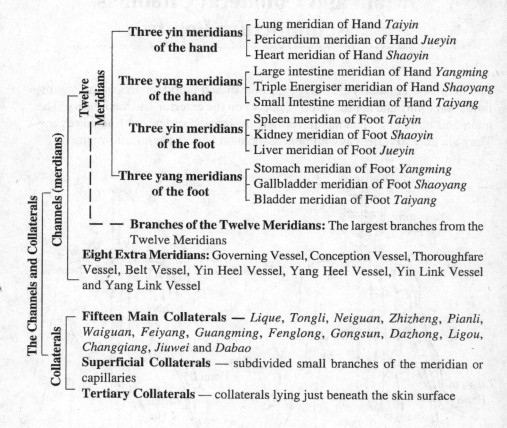

The Channels and Collaterals

Channels (merdians)

Twelve Meridians

Three yin meridians of the hand
- Lung meridian of Hand *Taiyin*
- Pericardium meridian of Hand *Jueyin*
- Heart meridian of Hand *Shaoyin*

Three yang meridians of the hand
- Large intestine meridian of Hand *Yangming*
- Triple Energiser meridian of Hand *Shaoyang*
- Small Intestine meridian of Hand *Taiyang*

Three yin meridians of the foot
- Spleen meridian of Foot *Taiyin*
- Kidney meridian of Foot *Shaoyin*
- Liver meridian of Foot *Jueyin*

Three yang meridians of the foot
- Stomach meridian of Foot *Yangming*
- Gallbladder meridian of Foot *Shaoyang*
- Bladder meridian of Foot *Taiyang*

Branches of the Twelve Meridians: The largest branches from the Twelve Meridians

Eight Extra Meridians: Governing Vessel, Conception Vessel, Thoroughfare Vessel, Belt Vessel, Yin Heel Vessel, Yang Heel Vessel, Yin Link Vessel and Yang Link Vessel

Collaterals

Fifteen Main Collaterals — *Lique, Tongli, Neiguan, Zhizheng, Pianli, Waiguan, Feiyang, Guangming, Fenglong, Gongsun, Dazhong, Ligou, Changqiang, Jiuwei* and *Dabao*

Superficial Collaterals — subdivided small branches of the meridian or capillaries

Tertiary Collaterals — collaterals lying just beneath the skin surface

Twelve Meridians: Also known as twelve regular meridians, each meridian corresponds to a *zang* or *fu* organ

Eight Extra Meridians: No direct link to the *zang* and *fu* organs. They are supplementary to the twelve regular meridians

Fifteen Main Collaterals: The larger of the collaterals in the body

Branches of the Twelve Meridians: Supplementary passage to the twelve regular meridians for the flow of qi in the meridians

Main and collateral channels and acupoints

The main and collateral channels transport qi and blood, connect the organs, limbs and joints and are the interface between the exterior and the interior throughout the body. The main and collateral channels have their designated order and related organs. They are able to reflect any ailment associated with the relevant organs.

An acupoint is a node where bundles of nervous tissue intersect. There are 720 acupoints in the human body, of which 108 are vital acupoints. Certain ailments may be treated via the stimulation of acupoints.

Commonly used acupoints:

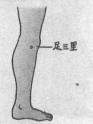

Zusanli Acupoint:
Treats indigestion, abdominal pains, diarrhoea, gastric ailments and high blood pressure.

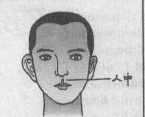

Renzhong Acupoint:
Treats coma/unconsciousness. Treats swollen faces and backaches as well.

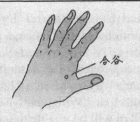

Hegu Acupoint:
The acupoint used to treat facial ailments. It also relieves headaches, toothaches, sore throats, colds, fevers etc.

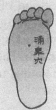

Tongquan point:
Treats headache, shock, partial paralysis, heat strokes, ringing in the ear, kidney infections, female ailments and diseases of the reproductive system.

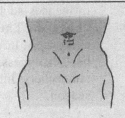

Mingmen point:
Treats impotency, low sperm count, weak limbs, deficiency of yang in the kidneys, backaches, ear diseases etc.

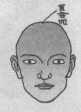

Baihui point:
Treats headaches, dizziness, insomnia, neuroses, stroke and loss of speech, low blood pressure etc

Endogenous and Exogenous Factors

Endogenous Factors

Endogenous factors refer to excessive emotional changes. Traditional Chinese medicine recognises seven types of emotions, which will be addressed in a later chapter.

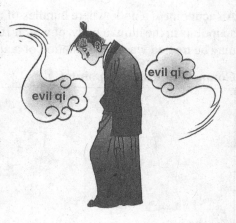

Health is affected by a person's emotional state. Hence, a person who is mentally distressed will be more susceptible to the assault of 'evil qi'. That's why traditional Chinese medicine holds that, "With positive qi in the body, evil qi will be unable to wreak havoc".

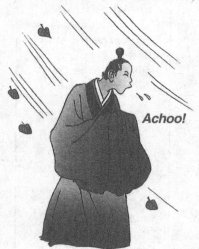

Achoo!

Exogenous Factors

Exogenous factors refer to environmental influences such as weather and climatic changes. There are six recognised atmospheric influences: wind, cold, summer heat, dampness, dryness and fire. These six atmospheric influences are unique to each season.

Sudden weather changes will cause the six atmospheric influences to go out of sync, as when the weather unexpectedly turns cold during spring or warm during winter. As the human body fails to cope with the sudden weather change, various ailments will arise.

Wind occurs mostly in springtime although all the four seasons have their windy spells. Wind is the main culprit behind many ailments. As wind is mobile, evil qi like cold, dryness, dampness and heat will penetrate the human body to cause problems like colds and rheumatism.

Cold occurs during winter when air temperature decreases. Cold is evil yin which can harm yang. When the body is affected by cold, symptoms like fever, lack of perspiration and headache will manifest.

Summer heat during the hot summer season may cause dizzy spells, cold sweat and cold hands and feet. They are symptoms of heatstroke.

Dampness is caused by increased humidity in the air. In rainy seasons, the ground becomes damp. People fall ill easily.

Dryness occurs in autumn when humidity is low. Dryness causes dry throat and mouth, among other ailments.

Fire is caused by heat. Wind, cold, summer heat and dryness may all lead to fire. Symptoms include high fevers, a ruddy complexion, emotional distress, thirst, etc.

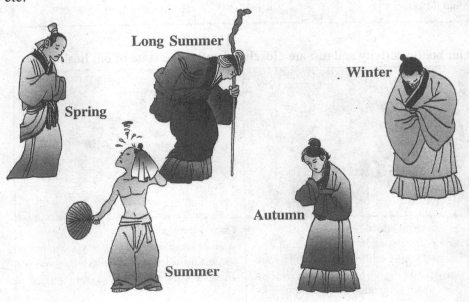

Neither Endogenous Nor Exogenous

As the saying goes, "We are what we eat". Our diet is also one of the prime causes of many ailments.

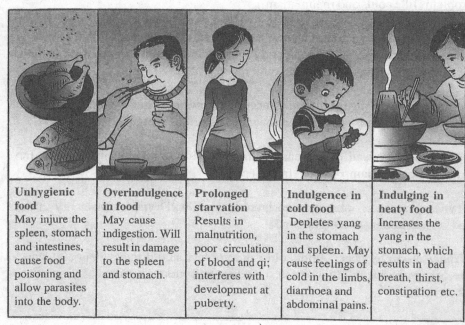

Unhygienic food	Overindulgence in food	Prolonged starvation	Indulgence in cold food	Indulging in heaty food
May injure the spleen, stomach and intestines, cause food poisoning and allow parasites into the body.	May cause indigestion. Will result in damage to the spleen and stomach.	Results in malnutrition, poor circulation of blood and qi; interferes with development at puberty.	Depletes yang in the stomach and spleen. May cause feelings of cold in the limbs, diarrhoea and abdominal pains.	Increases the yang in the stomach, which results in bad breath, thirst, constipation etc.

Our bodily activity and rest are closely related to the state of our health.

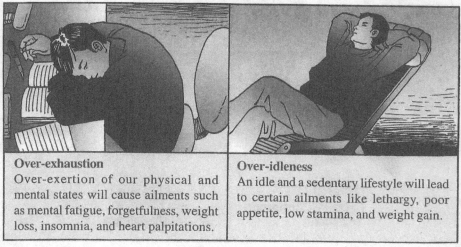

Over-exhaustion	Over-idleness
Over-exertion of our physical and mental states will cause ailments such as mental fatigue, forgetfulness, weight loss, insomnia, and heart palpitations.	An idle and a sedentary lifestyle will lead to certain ailments like lethargy, poor appetite, low stamina, and weight gain.

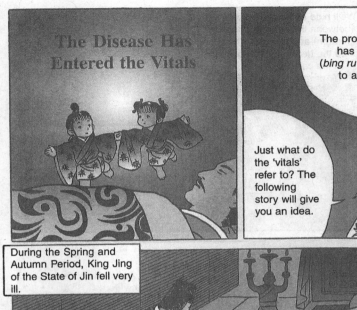

The Disease Has Entered the Vitals

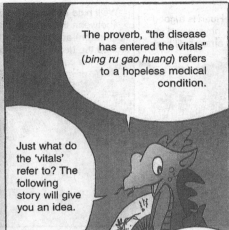

The proverb, "the disease has entered the vitals" (*bing ru gao huang*) refers to a hopeless medical condition.

Just what do the 'vitals' refer to? The following story will give you an idea.

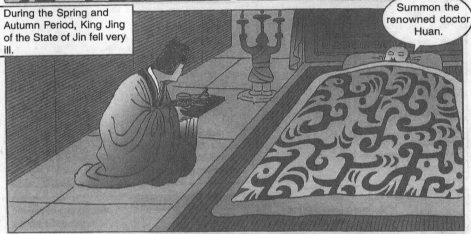

During the Spring and Autumn Period, King Jing of the State of Jin fell very ill.

Summon the renowned doctor Huan.

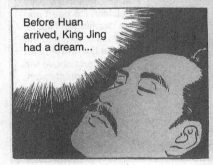

Before Huan arrived, King Jing had a dream...

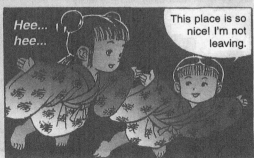

Hee... hee...

This place is so nice! I'm not leaving.

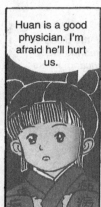

Huan is a good physician. I'm afraid he'll hurt us.

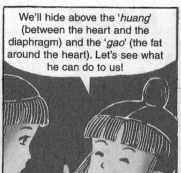

We'll hide above the '*huang*' (between the heart and the diaphragm) and the '*gao*' (the fat around the heart). Let's see what he can do to us!

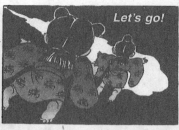

Let's go!

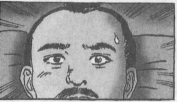

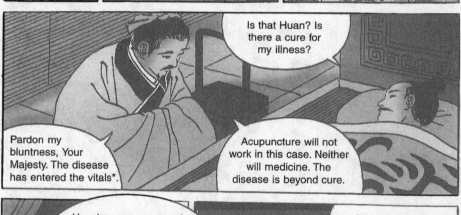

Is that Huan? Is there a cure for my illness?

Pardon my bluntness, Your Majesty. The disease has entered the vitals*.

Acupuncture will not work in this case. Neither will medicine. The disease is beyond cure.

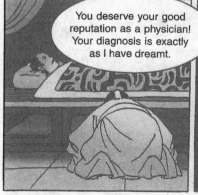

You deserve your good reputation as a physician! Your diagnosis is exactly as I have dreamt.

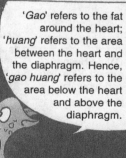

'*Gao*' refers to the fat around the heart; '*huang*' refers to the area between the heart and the diaphragm. Hence, '*gao huang*' refers to the area below the heart and above the diaphragm.

* bing ru gao huang

How To Prevent Diseases

Illness is caused by evil qi. Falling ill is like a battle between good and evil. Hence, to prevent illnesses, we need to build up the positive energy in our bodies to prevent the invasion of negative energy.

Cultivating positive energy

Insufficient positive energy is one of the major causes of diseases. Cultivating positive energy will strengthen the constitution and increase resistance level, maintain good health and prolong life. How do we cultivate positive energy? Here are a few ways:

1. Adapt to the ways of nature: The human body and nature share a close relationship, hence the need for the body to be in harmony with nature. "Yang is strong in spring and summer; yin is built in autumn and winter". This knowledge should make it difficult for diseases to invade us.

2. Acknowledge the importance of mental well-being: Keep a happy and cheerful disposition. Our physical body is affected by our mental health. Staying happy will keep us healthy.

3. Pay attention to diet and lifestyle: A balanced diet and regular lifestyle with appropriate rest and activity will leave one with abundant energy and a healthy body.

4. Strengthen the physique: Exercises like *qigong*, *taijiquan* and *wushu* are ways to boost blood circulation, strengthen muscles and bone and improve strength.

5. Preventive aids: Innoculation and moderate ingestion of vitamins and herbal tonics will also help build immunity and boost resistance to pathogens.

Combating evil qi

When evil qi enters the body, one falls ill. Avoidance of evil qi will reduce the occurrence of ailments.

Below are ways to prevent or bring ailments under control:

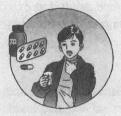

1. The use of drugs to destroy agents of diseases: Application of medicated creams, cleansing and disinfection of infected areas, ingestion of drugs to destroy the cause of diseases.

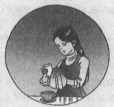

2. Personal hygiene: Pathogens often lurk in our surroundings. Food hygiene, clean water and surroundings will prevent viruses and bacteria from multiplying.

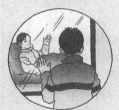

3. Avoiding sources of infection: Avoid direct contact with someone who is infectious to prevent the disease from spreading.

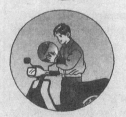

4. Prevention of accidents and injuries: The immunity level will drop when hurt or injured, hence the chances of catching a disease will increase.

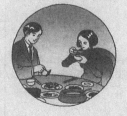

5. Proper preparation and handling of food: We are what we eat. Eating is a daily activity. Food gives our body the energy to carry out our daily activities. But if the food is not prepared or handled properly, it may cause illness instead.

Traditional Chinese Medical Science (The Skill of Qi And Huang)
Traditional Chinese medical science is also known as The Skill of Qi and Huang. Qi and Huang refer to two persons — Huang Di (Yellow Emperor) and Qi Bo. Huang Di is the ancestor of the Chinese people. Legend has it that he founded Chinese traditional medicine. Qi Bo, learned in medical science, was a subject of Huang Di. As they were the earliest proponents of Chinese medical theories which laid the foundation for Chinese medicine, people began to use 'Qi Huang' to refer to Chinese medical science.

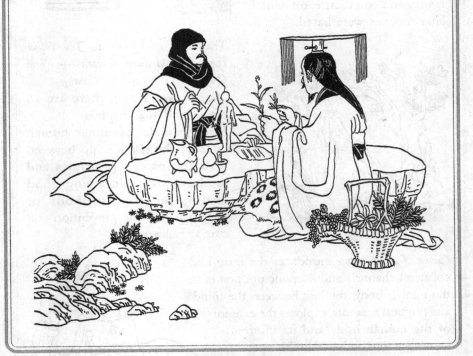

The Treasure of Chinese Medical Science - *The Yellow Emperor's Medicine Classic*

Any discourse on Chinese medical science will inevitably mention *The Yellow Emperor's Medicine Classic.*

Compiled during the Warring States Period, this work is a collection of the medical anecdotes and theories of many ancient physicians.

The famous *Yellow Emperor's Medicine Classic* was the earliest compilation which explained human physiology, ailments and their treatments, diagnosis, prevention and the maintenance of good health through an understanding of yin-yang and the five elements. It laid the foundations of Chinese traditional medicine on which later theories were based.

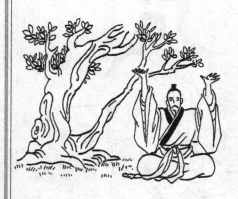

There are two parts to *The Yellow Emperor's Medicine Classic* — *Plain Questions* and *Canon of Acupuncture.* In all, there are 18 scrolls and 162 chapters.

Plain Questions examines human puberty, the relationship between man and nature, principles and methods of maintaining good health, the four methods of diagnosis and the prevention and cure of ailments.

Canon of Acupuncture introduces the main and collateral channels and acupuncture points in the human body, the link between the mind and physical ailments, explores the exterior of the human body and its internal organs, various body and health types, acupuncture etc.

Methods of Diagnosis in Traditional Chinese Medicine

Traditional Chinese medicine has its own unique diagnostic methods. Chinese medical practice has no use for stethoscopes, X-ray machines or other diagnostic equipment. Instead, observation, auscultation and olfaction, interrogation and pulse taking are employed to diagnose diseases.

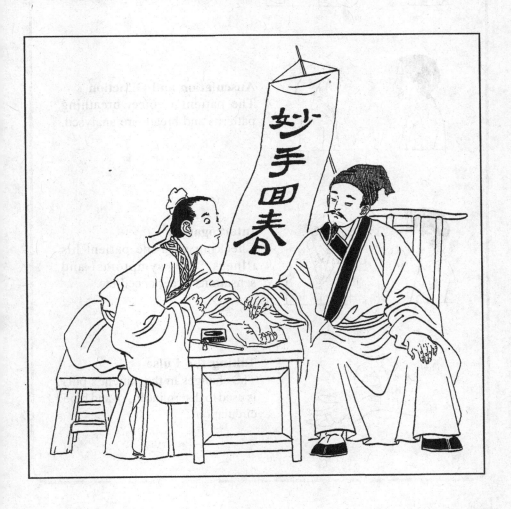

The Four Diagnoses

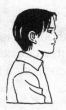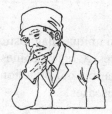

Observation
Inspection of the patient's general well-being, colour of complexion etc.

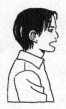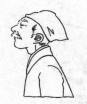

Ausculation and Olfaction
The patient's voice, breathing patterns and breath are analysed.

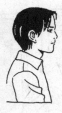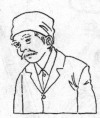

Interrogation
Checking with the patient his illness, the symptoms and sensations experienced etc.

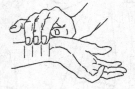

Taking the Pulse
The changes in the patient's pulse is used to determine his qi and blood circulation.

Diagnosis Through Observation

A person's complexion and his vital organs share a close relationship. Any changes in the blood and qi circulation in the vitals will be reflected in a person's physical appearance, including observing the person's energy level and the colour of his face and tongue.

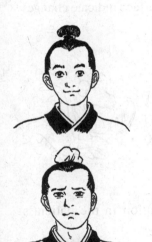

Observing the patient's energy level

Observation of the patient's vitality, expression in his eyes, facial expression etc. A person's energy may be classified into the following types:

Vigour and vitality present:
Energetic, lively eyes, a bright countenance, etc. They indicate a mild case of illness where the vital energy has not been diminished. It signals a quick recovery.

Vigour and vitality absent:
Listless, lethargic, dull eyes, absentmindedness, slowed responses etc. The patient is deficient in vital energy and seriously ill.

Observing the patient's complexion

When a person falls ill, his complexion will take on an unusual colour. This is known as the pathogeny of complexion. In all, there are five colours.

Blue	Caused by wind and cold, marked by a sensation of pain.
Yellow	Caused by dampness, marked by deficiency of vital energy and lowering of body resistance.
Red	Caused by heat.
White	Caused by deficiency in vital energy and poor blood circulation.
Black	Caused by cold, pain, fluid retention and blood clots.

Observing the tongue

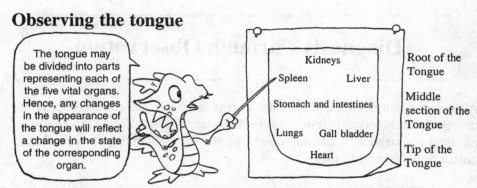

The tongue may be divided into parts representing each of the five vital organs. Hence, any changes in the appearance of the tongue will reflect a change in the state of the corresponding organ.

Kidneys	Root of the Tongue
Spleen Liver	
Stomach and intestines	Middle section of the Tongue
Lungs Gall bladder	
Heart	Tip of the Tongue

The colour and appearance of the coating of the tongue surface indicate changes in the patient's condition:

Colour of the coating:
White ⇄ Yellow ⇄ Grey ⇄ Black

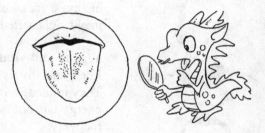

Appearance of the coating:
Moist ⇄ Dry ⇄ Dry and black
⇄ Dry and prickly
Thin ⇄ Thick
Present ⇄ Absent

The progression from left to right indicates deterioration in the patient's condition, and vice versa.

The colour, degree of plumpness and softness of the tongue are also important. Here are some conditions and what they might mean.

A whitish tongue	Indicates deficiency in vital energy and blood.
A deep red tongue	Indicates presence of heat.
A plump tongue	Usually related to presence of phlegm, dampness, heat and toxins.
A thin and shrunken tongue	Usually suggests deficiency in vital energy and blood, or interior heat.
A stiff tongue	Usually seen in exogenic diseases, may indicate the possibility of stroke.
A soft and curled tongue	Usually suggests deficiency in vital energy and blood.

Observing the Five Sense Organs and hair

The condition of one's ears, eyes, lips, nose, hair and skin also reflect the body's state of health. Some examples are listed below:

Swollen eyes	Usually caused by water retention.
Dry eyes	Usually caused by deficiency of blood in the liver.
Swollen and red eyes	Usually caused by wind-heat.
Blocked nose; clear mucus	Usually caused by wind-cold.
Blocked nose; thick yellow mucus	Usually caused by wind-heat.
Dry and thin outer ear	Asthenia (abnormal loss of strength) of kidney.
Dark, red lips	Caused by cold factors, usually seen in weak lungs.
Pale lips	Usually caused by deficiency of blood.
Dark red and dry lips	Usually caused by febrile factors, characterised by a high fever.
Dry, cracked lips	Insufficient bodily fluids.
Dry skin	Insufficient bodily fluids; exhaustion of internal vital essences and blood.
Dry and prickly skin	Usually caused by atrophy of the lungs.
Black, thick and lustrous hair	Healthy kidneys, sufficient blood and vital energy.
Brown, sparse and dry hair	Deficiency of vital essence and blood, usually seen after a major illness.
Dry and brittle hair	Heat in the blood and deficiency of yin.
Curly and oily hair	Usually caused by heat in the blood.
Greying of hair among youths	Caused by worry and anxiety; accumulation of pathogenic heat in blood.
Thinning of hair among youths	Asthenia of kidneys or pathogenic heat in blood.
Slow growth of hair; thin and brown hair	Usually caused by hereditary factors and a weak constitution.

Observing A Child's Index Finger

This type of diagnosis is suitable for children under the age of three. The channels and collaterals on the inside of the child's index finger are examined. The diagnosis is based on the observation of the meridian phenomena and colour.

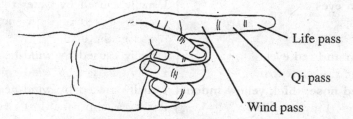

- Life pass
- Qi pass
- Wind pass

Diagram of the Index Finger

During the finger diagnosis, the child should be carried in a well-lit place where the physician will use his left hand to keep the tip of the child's index finger in place. He will rub the child's index finger from its tip towards the palm with his right hand a few times until the branches of channels show for inspection.

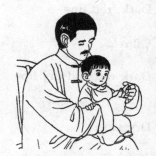

Collaterals show in the wind point zone	The disease is within the collaterals; the condition is not serious.
Collaterals show in the qi point zone.	The disease has attacked the channels; condition is quite serious.
Collaterals are evident in all three zones.	The disease has attacked the viscera; condition is serious.
Collaterals show beyond the fingertip.	The situation is very grave.
Collaterals show clearly.	The disease is an exogenous one affecting the exterior of the body.
Collaterals are not obvious.	The disease is an endogenous one affecting the internal organs.
Collaterals are reddish.	Usually caused by cold factors.
Collaterals are purplish.	Usually caused by febrile factors.
Collaterals are greenish.	Caused by wind, cold, or pain.
Collaterals are pale and thin.	Usually caused by cold factors.
Collaterals are dull and thick.	Excess syndrome.

Auscultatory and Olfactory Diagnosis

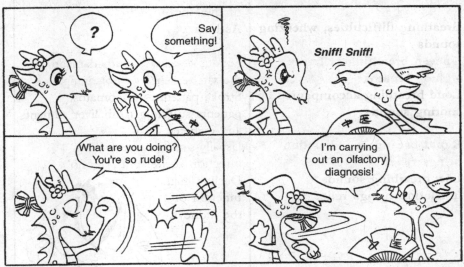

Diagnosis through auscultation and olfaction involves listening to the patient's tone of voice, breathing patterns and taking a sniff of the patient's breath. The following tables show some of the conditions that may occur and what they mean.

Listening to the patient's voice

Strong, loud voice	Presence of yang, heat.
Feeble, broken voice	Presence of yin, cold. Shows as deficient vital energy and lowered resistance.
Hoarseness or loss of voice due to recent illness	Caused by febrile factors, usually the result of external colds and heat.
Hoarseness or loss of voice due to prolonged illness	Lack of energy and reduced resistance; weakness of the lungs and kidneys.
Deep coughs, clear phlegm	Wind-cold has attacked the lungs.
Sudden coughing, thick and yellow phlegm	Excess heat in the lungs.
Phlegmy cough	Presence of phlegm.

Listening to the patient's breathing

Strong and heavy breathing	Caused by febrile factors, excess pathogenic internal heat.
Weak, short breaths	Caused by deficiency in the function of the lungs.
Breathing difficulties, wheezing sounds	Asthma.
Uneven breathing or heavy sighing breaths	Serious condition, with damage to the vital essence or poisoning.
Loud breathing accompanied by snoring sounds	Stroke patients and comatose patients suffering from liver ailments and diabetes.
Rapid breathing, exhalation brings relief	Usually seen in cases of lung infection or phlegm-retention.
Low breathing sounds, inhalation brings relief	Decline in the function of the kidneys. 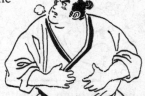

Inspection through smell

Bad breath	Poor digestion, heat in the stomach or poor oral hygiene.
Sourish breath	Undigested food in one's system.
Decaying breath	Stomach ulcer and sores.
Body odour	Caused by pathogenic dampness-heat.
Nose emits odour, runny nose	Heat in the lungs or pathogenic dampness-heat accumulated in the spleen and the stomach.

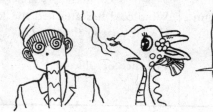

Doctor, I think I have bad breath. Please check for me.

Diagnosis Through Interrogation

This involves asking the patient about his illness, the symptoms and how he feels. Through the patient's answers, a diagnosis is made. It is therefore a very important part of a diagnosis.

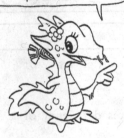

Diagnosis through interrogation is very comprehensive. It's even been made into a ditty that lists 10 commonly asked questions.

"First, you ask about chills and fever.
Next, you move to perspiration.
Third, you ask about general pains and headaches.
Fourth, you ask about urination and defecation.
Fifth, you ask about the appetite.
Next, you ask about sensations in the chest and abdomen.
The seventh question concerns hearing and sight.
The eighth question touches on one's sleep pattern.
The ninth question checks past medical history and the tenth inquires of the causes of the new disease.
In female adult patients, check on their menstrual cycle.
In young patients, it will be measles."

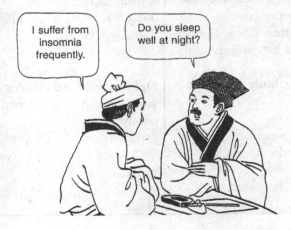

I suffer from insomnia frequently.

Do you sleep well at night?

35

Tables showing some possible conditions and what they mean:

Chills and fever	
Feeling feverish in the morning	Deficiency of gallbladder energy.
Feeling feverish in the afternoon	Deficiency of yin, dampness-heat.
Feverish without feeling cold	Excess yang nature, usually seen in acute diseases.
Feeling chilly without having a fever	Deficiency of yang nature, usually seen in chronic diseases.
The limbs feel cold	Deficiency of yang.
Heat in the abdomen and chest	Accumulated internal heat.
The whole body is feverish and is afraid of cold	Usually caused by febrile factors.

Perspiration	
Perspiration before bedtime which stops on waking (night sweat)	Usually indicates deficiency of yin.
Perspiring easily during the day (spontaneous sweating)	Usually indicates deficiency of yang.
Afraid of cold, perspiration, cold limbs (cold sweat)	Usually indicates deficiency of yang.
Perspiration followed by shivering	Body battling an infectious disease.
Perspiration only on the forehead (Children often perspire on the forehead when they sleep. If no other symptoms are present, this is not a sign of illness.)	Usually indicates heat in the abdomen and pathogenic dampness-heat.
Only half of the body perspires	Deficiency of gallbladder energy and blood. A sign of partial paralysis.
Perspiration on the chest	Deficiency of yin of the heart.
Perspiration of the hands and feet	Deficiency of yin and excess of yang.
Perspiration of the palms	Usually caused by anxiety and nervousness.

Appetite	
Preference for cold drinks when thirsty	Endogenous heat.
Preference for warm drinks when thirsty	Endogenous cold.
Low consumption of water despite being thirsty	Pathogenic dampness-heat in the spleen and stomach.
Dulled sense of taste	Asthenia of the spleen and stomach.
Bitter taste in mouth	Heat in the liver and gallbladder.
Sour taste in mouth	Retention of undigested food in the stomach and intestines.
Sweet taste in mouth	Pathogenic dampness-heat in the spleen and stomach.
Partiality in limited variety of food	Usually caused by presence of parasites.
Gets hungry easily	Heat in the stomach or incomplete digestion.
Bloating after a meal	Asthenia of spleen and blockage of gallbladder.
Poor appetite, bloated stomach, sour breath	Retention of undigested food in the stomach and intestines, poor digestion.
Frequent micturition, constant intake of fluid, thirst	Thirst relief (diabetes).

Ears and eyes	
Sound in the ear	Deficiency of the liver and kidney.
Pain in the ear	Infection of the inner ear.
Deafness in the ear	Deficiency of the kidney, infectious febrile disease.
Echoes in the ear	Deficiency of the kidney or pathogenic wind.
Blurred vision, night blindness	Deficiency of the liver.
Swollen and red eyes	Heat in the liver.

General pains and headaches	
Nagging headache	Usually caused by exogenous heat.
Sporadic headache	Usually caused by internal injury.
Headache in the morning	Usually a deficiency of vital energy.
Headache in the afternoon	Usually a deficiency of blood.
Headache in the day	Deficiency of yang.
Headache in the evening	Deficiency of yin.
Feverish and aching body	Endogenous heat.
Backache	Deficiency of the kidney.
Sharp pain in the back	Stagnation of vital energy and stasis of blood.
Stuffy chest, shortness of breath, lethargy	Deficiency of vital energy.
Stuffy chest, long sighs	Stagnation of vital energy.
Pain on both sides of the rib cage	Stagnation of vital energy in the liver.
Abdominal pain; aversion to touch, inclination towards cold drinks, sharp abdominal pain after meals	Excess heat.
Abdominal pain; comfort from massage, loose stools	Deficiency of yang in the spleen and stomach.
Joints ache during rainy days	Caused by dampness-cold.
Swelling and pain	Depression, stagnation of digestion in the stomach, blocked respiratory system.
Sharp pain	Stasis of blood, stagnation of vital energy
Angina (chest pains)	Blood stasis, parasites, gallstones.
Nagging, dull pain	Poor blood and vital energy circulation; endogenous yin and cold.
Aches	Dampness in the joints; poor blood and vital energy circulation.
Aversion to cold; excruciating pain	Usually caused by cold factors.
Aversion to heat; redness and swelling	Usually caused by heat factors.
Sudden pain	Syndrome of excess due to exogenous factors.
Prolonged pain	Deficiency of yin.

Urination and defecation

Constipation	Heat, sluggish vital energy or blood exhaustion.
Hard stools	Deficiency of middle-energiser energy or poor liver function.
Whitish stools	Jaundice or deficiency of cold in large intestines.
Black stools	Internal bleeding.
Red stools	Blood in the stools or dysentery.
Clear urine	Caused by cold factors.
Dark yellow urine	Caused by heat factors.
Pain during urination	Caused by stranguria (spasm of the urethra and bladder).
Turbid (cloudy) urine	Febrile diseases caused by dampness and heat.
Incontinence	Deficiency of vital energy and strokes.
Difficulty in passing urine	Caused by dampness-heat harm or damage to the body fluids.

Menstruation (Gynaecology)

Early period, high volume, blood is bright red	Heat in the blood.
Period delayed, low volume, pale colour, pain in the lower abdomen	Interior cold.
Irregular periods	Stagnation of the liver energy or asthenia of the spleen and kidneys, or blockage due to blood clot.
Absence of menstruation	Deficiency of vital energy and low blood volume; stagnation of the vital energy and blood stasis.
Uterine bleeding	Heat in the blood, Deficiency of the vital energy.

Sleep patterns	
Insomnia	Over-anxiety, deficiency of the heart and spleen.
Inability to sleep combined with thirst and feeling of vexation	Usually indicates deficiency of the yin of the heart.
Inability to sleep combined with feeling of panic	Usually indicates deficiency of the gallbladder energy.
Inability to sleep combined with dizziness and panic	Usually indicates deficiency of blood in the heart and spleen.
Inability to sleep combined with dizziness and heavy head	Usually indicates an excess of yang of the liver.
Inability to sleep combined with fullness of the stomach	Usually caused by lack of coordination of the spleen, resulting in nausea and vomiting.
Wakes up easily	Usually indicates lack of vital energy of the heart and the gallbladder, excess heat in the heart.
Wakes up early	Usually indicates deficiency of vital energy.
Unable to fall asleep	Anxiety, insufficient vital energy.
Sleep disturbed by many dreams	Deficiency of yin of the liver and kidneys, imbalance of yin and yang.
Constant sleepiness, lethargy	Usually indicates asthenia of the spleen or accumulation of dampness.

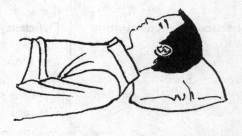

Diagnosis Through Pulse Taking and Palpation

The changes in one's pulse are used to determine the level of qi and blood in one's body.

The human wrist can be divided into three sections: inch, bar and cubit. Each section corresponds to different internal organs.

In general, traditional Chinese medicine uses the entrance to the pulse, ie. the inch section. As it is where the Hand *Taiyin* lung channel passes through, bearing in mind that the lungs are the part of the viscera that store qi, blood and nutrients, and are crucial to the limbs and bones, this section will reveal the state of the viscera, channels and collaterals, qi and blood etc.

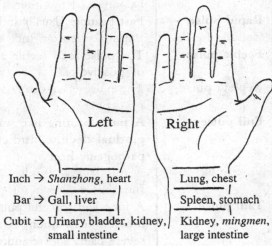

Inch → *Shanzhong*, heart   Lung, chest

Bar → Gall, liver   Spleen, stomach

Cubit → Urinary bladder, kidney, small intestine   Kidney, *mingmen*, large intestine

Diagram of Palms

When a person is in good health, the pulse is slow and steady, rhythmic and strong. A rapid or a very slow pulse will indicate presence of disease.
If a patient is very ill, but the pulse is calm and strong, it indicates a chance of recovery. But if the pulse is fine and faint, almost imperceptible, it is a portent of grave consequences.

There are many types of pulse, such as floating pulse, deep pulse, full pulse, fine pulse, feeble pulse, replete pulse and others. The differences are very subtle. Hence diagnosis through pulse taking is not easy to master.

An overview of various types of pulse

Floating pulse	Can be felt by a light touch. It grows faint on hard pressure and can be likened to a floating log. Usually seen in early stages of diseases caused by exogenous factors.
Deep pulse	Can only be felt by applying pressure. Usually seen in many various chronic diseases. Indicates that the disease has attacked the internal organs.
Rapid pulse	Fast beating. Usually indicates the presence of heat.
Retarded pulse	Pulse beat is slow. Indicates diseases of a cold nature.
Feeble pulse	The pulse feels feeble and faint. Indicates deficiency of positive qi.
Replete pulse	The pulse is vigorous and forceful. Indicates excess syndrome.
Full pulse	A pulse beating like waves with forceful rising and gradual decline. Indicates presence of excessive pathogenic heat.
Fine pulse	A thin, thready pulse. Faint yet always perceptible. Indicates deficiency of yin and blood.
Taut pulse	A long and forceful pulse that feels like a string on a musical instrument. Usually seen in liver trouble, severe pains and retention of phlegm.
Tense pulse	A fast and strong pulse that feels like a tightly stretched cord. Indicates presence of cold or pain.
Knotted pulse	A pulse pausing at irregular intervals. Usually seen in cases of stagnation of qi or blood, phlegm due to cold.
Intermittent pulse	A slow and weak pulse pausing at regular intervals. Indicates severely weakened viscera, deficiency of the qi and blood, severe trauma or terror.
Running pulse	A rapid pulse with irregular intermittence. Usually seen in cases of excessive heat, stagnation of qi and blood, retention of phlegm or indigestion.
Slippery pulse	A smooth pulse running like beads rolling on a plate. Usually seen in cases of phlegm retention.
Hesitant pulse	An uneven pulse. Usually caused by loss or stagnation of qi and blood.

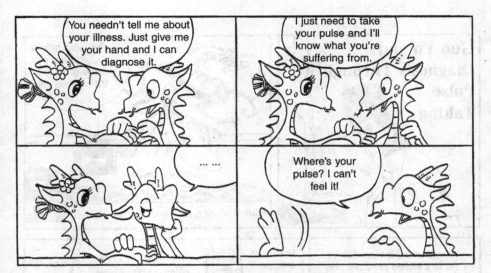

It is an exaggeration to say that feeling the pulse will be able to tell one what the patient is suffering from. Diagnosis cannot be based on pulse taking alone. The four methods of diagnosis are not self-contained. During a consultation, all four methods of diagnosis have to be exercised before a comprehensive and accurate diagnosis can be made.

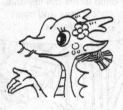

Wang Shuhe and the *Pulse Classic*

Wang Shuhe (180–270 AD) was a famous physician from the Western Jin state. He studied sphygmology*. He compiled the various documents on sphygmology from generations before him and his own experience in this area of medicine into a book known as the *Pulse Classic*.

The *Pulse Classic* categorised pulse conditions into 24 types. They still form the basis for methods of diagnosis in traditional Chinese medicine to date. The book established the study of the entrance of the pulse and clearly defined the inch, bar and cubit sections.

The *Pulse Classic* was China's earliest work on sphygmology and was highly regarded by later physicians. Its influence in the medical field was extensive, later spreading to China, Korea, the Arab world and Europe.

* *The study of the pulse.*

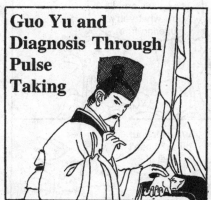

Guo Yu and Diagnosis Through Pulse Taking

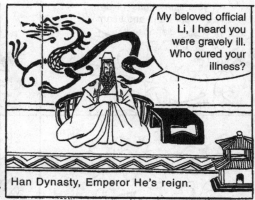

My beloved official Li, I heard you were gravely ill. Who cured your illness?

Han Dynasty, Emperor He's reign.

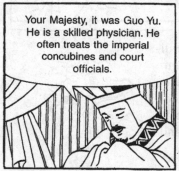

Your Majesty, it was Guo Yu. He is a skilled physician. He often treats the imperial concubines and court officials.

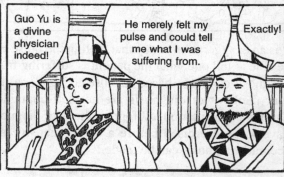

Guo Yu is a divine physician indeed!

He merely felt my pulse and could tell me what I was suffering from.

Exactly!

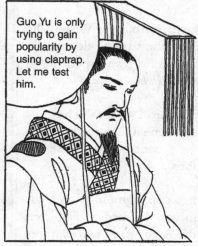

Guo Yu is only trying to gain popularity by using claptrap. Let me test him.

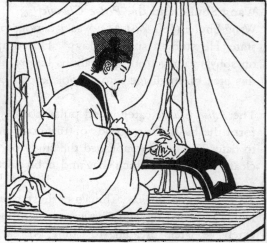

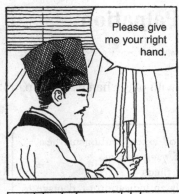

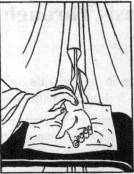

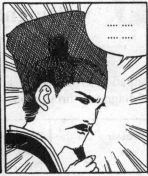

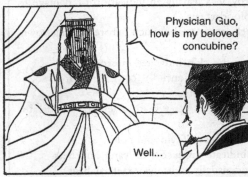

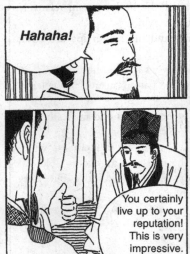

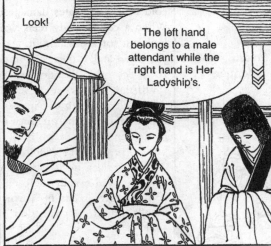

Diagnosis Through Palpation

Palpation involves pressing on the patient's body with one's hands. It is a part of diagnosis through pulse feeling and palpation.

Pressing on the skin	Warm skin indicates the presence of excess pathogenic heat. Cold skin indicates a deficiency of yang and qi. Dry skin indicates a deficiency of fluids. If the skin feels thorny, it is usually an indication of damage to the yin or internal blood stasis. If the skin initially feels warm to the touch before cooling down, the heat is external. A gradual warming of the skin indicates internal heat.
Pressing on swellings	When the swelling remains dented after being pressed, it indicates the presence of oedema. When the swelling pops back after being pressed, it indicates the presence of air.
Pressing on the limbs	Cold limbs indicate an excess of yin and cold. Warm limbs usually indicate an excess of yang and heat. A warm back of hand usually indicates external heat. A warm palm where other parts of the body remain relatively cold usually indicates damage to the yin. When a child's body feels warm and his fingertips are cold, look out for a possible fit.
Pressing on the abdomen	A painful and swollen abdomen suggests exogenous causes. A swollen but soft abdomen with no pain indicates a deficiency syndrome. A swollen abdomen which rises when pressed and makes hollow sounds indicates the presence of excess air. A swollen abdomen which shows wave-like movements when pressed on both sides indicates the presence of excess fluid. A hard swelling in the abdomen which doesn't move and hurts when pressed usually indicates blood stasis. A swelling that has no form, is painless and moves around usually indicates a stagnation of qi.

Diagnosis Through the Analysis of Excreta

Stools and urine are waste products from the human body. They offer telling signs of a person's state of health. In general, stools are yellowish brown. But if they remain in the intestines for too long, they'll turn a darker colour and become drier. In diarrhoea, the stools are more yellowish as they have stayed in the intestines for only a short time.

Examination of stools and urine are commonly carried out in hospital checkups. They provide a basis for diagnosis. Examination of stools and urine involve the physical appearance, consistency, colour, degree of digestion, etc.

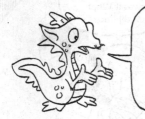

Examination of stool is not exactly a part of traditional Chinese medicine. But there have been records of tasting of stool in China to diagnose a patient. It's said that bitter stools indicate signs of recovery while sweet stools are bad news. Just how accurate and true is this? Well, no harm reading it up for fun.

The King of Yue Tastes Stool

During the Spring and Summer Period when the states of Yue and Wu were at war, the state of Yue lost and the king of Yue was held as a prisoner-of-war. The king of Yue took the humiliation in his stride. In order to gain the trust of the king of Wu, he tasted King Wu's stool when the latter fell ill and predicted a full recovery. True enough, the king of Wu got his health back and released the king of Yue. The king of Yue then returned to rebuild his country and eventually defeated the state of Wu.

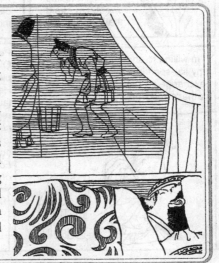

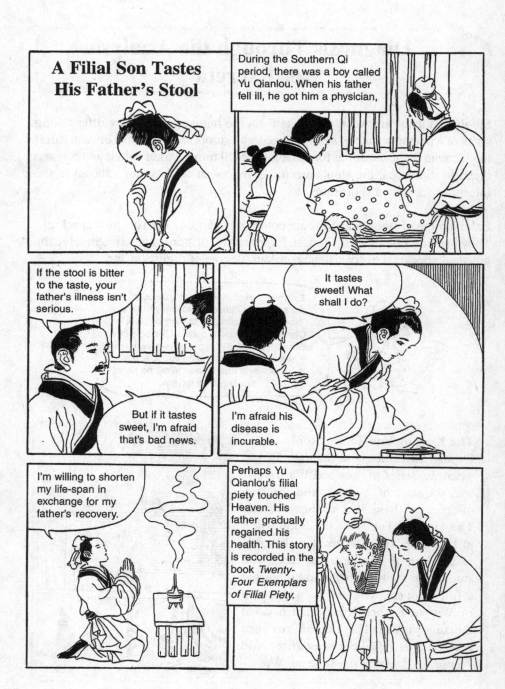

A Filial Son Tastes His Father's Stool

During the Southern Qi period, there was a boy called Yu Qianlou. When his father fell ill, he got him a physician,

If the stool is bitter to the taste, your father's illness isn't serious.

But if it tastes sweet, I'm afraid that's bad news.

It tastes sweet! What shall I do?

I'm afraid his disease is incurable.

I'm willing to shorten my life-span in exchange for my father's recovery.

Perhaps Yu Qianlou's filial piety touched Heaven. His father gradually regained his health. This story is recorded in the book *Twenty-Four Exemplars of Filial Piety*.

METHODS OF TREATMENT IN TRADITIONAL CHINESE MEDICINE

The methods of treatment in traditional Chinese medicine are many and diverse in nature. The commonly-seen ones are Chinese medicine, acupuncture and moxibustion, massage, diet therapy, *qigong* and mood therapy, though there are more unusual therapies, such as cupping, scraping and bloodletting. The methods of treatment used vary depending on the ailment and constitution of each patient.

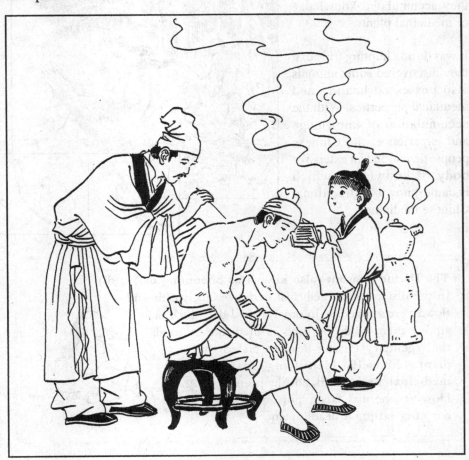

Method One — Chinese Medicines

Discovery of Chinese medicinal herbs

An ancient saying tells us: "The Divine Peasant tasted a hundred types of herbs to treat the diseases of the people." In their quest for survival, the forefathers of the Chinese people tasted countless wild fruit, seeds and plants. Over time, they learnt to distinguish the poisonous plants from the non-poisonous ones and discovered which ones had healing properties. In this way they accumulated knowledge of medicinal plants.

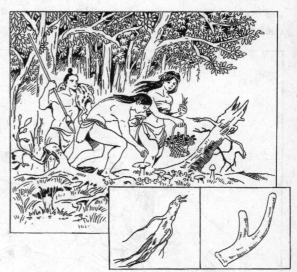

It was during hunting trips that they discovered some animals also possessed healing and medicinal properties. With the accumulation of knowledge and experience, the Chinese people developed an extensive body of knowledge which became known as traditional Chinese medicine.

The Divine Peasant (also known as Shennong or Yandi)
In the distant past, medicinal herbs, grains, weeds and flowers grew together. In order to find out which ones among them could be used as medicine or food, the legendary Divine Peasant tasted the plants himself, identifying many medicinal herbs and edible plants. However, he was fatally poisoned one day after tasting a deadly plant.

Types of Chinese medicines

Apart from the medicinal herbs we are familiar with, Chinese medicine also includes minerals and animal parts. China, with its vast land area, varied terrain and range of climatic conditions, is home to a wide variety of plants, animals and minerals. The definitive classic on Chinese medicines, the *Compendium of Materia Medica*, records 1892 types of medicines. Today, the number of possible medicines that can be found from these rich resources easily number in the thousands.

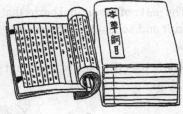

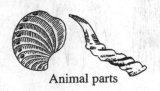
Animal parts

Minerals

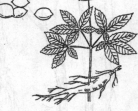
Medicinal herbs

Where medicinal herbs can be found

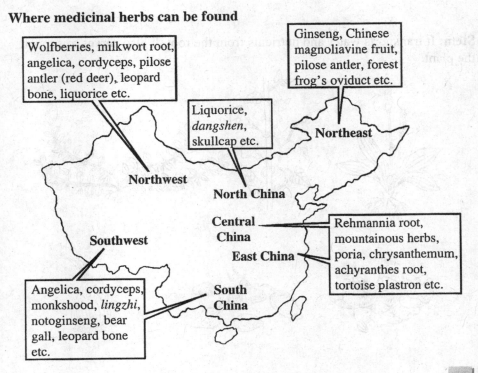

Wolfberries, milkwort root, angelica, cordyceps, pilose antler (red deer), leopard bone, liquorice etc.

Ginseng, Chinese magnoliavine fruit, pilose antler, forest frog's oviduct etc.

Liquorice, *dangshen*, skullcap etc.

Northeast

Northwest

North China

Central China

East China

Southwest

South China

Rehmannia root, mountainous herbs, poria, chrysanthemum, achyranthes root, tortoise plastron etc.

Angelica, cordyceps, monkshood, *lingzhi*, notoginseng, bear gall, leopard bone etc.

Medicinal herbs

The parts of medicinal herbs that are used include the root, bark, leaves, flowers, fruit and seed, cane and more.

Root: It is the part of the plant that absorbs nutrients and water from the soil and air.

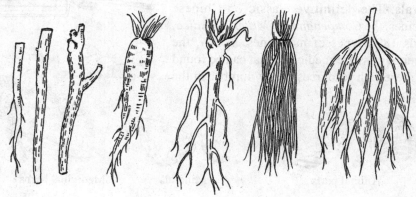

Stem: It transports water and nutrients from the root. It also serves to support the plant.

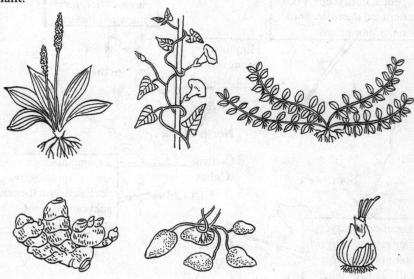

Leaf: The part where the plant makes food.

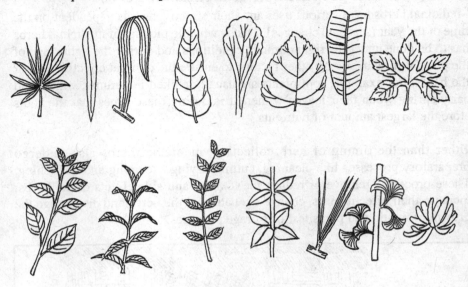

Flower: Mainly responsible for the reproduction of the plant.

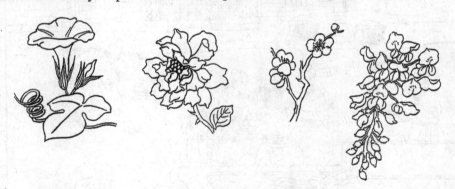

Fruit: A fertilized part of the plant with reproductive function.

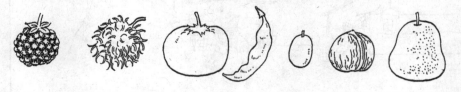

Collection and preparation of medicinal herbs

Medicinal herbs have various uses and their effectiveness is dependent on the time of the year (seasonal changes). That is why the picking of medicinal herbs has to be done under the right climatic conditions and during the right stage of the plant's growth, among other factors, to ensure the optimal effectiveness of the herbs. For example, root plants are usually picked in autumn, winter and early spring when their leaves wither. It is during these times that the roots store the largest amount of nutrients.

Other than the timing of herb collection, medicinal herbs also undergo preparatory processes like cleaning, cutting, frying, steaming and quenching. These processes remove or reduce the toxicity and side effects of the herbs; increase their effectiveness, change the nature of the herbs and discourage the growth of mould and parasites for storage purposes.

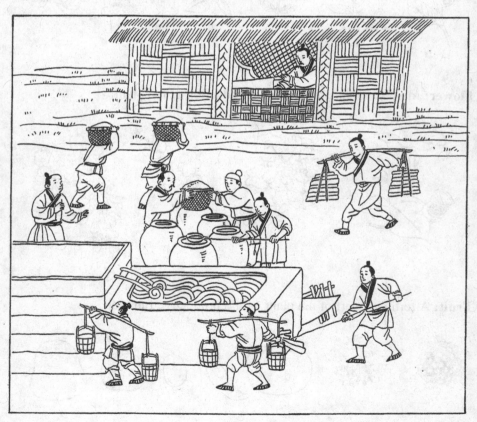

Some common medicinal herbs

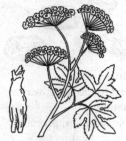

Angelica root:
Sweet and hot to the taste, warm in nature. Tonic for the qi and blood, moistens the intestines to ease constipation. Good for deficiency of blood, weak constitution, constipation and external injuries.

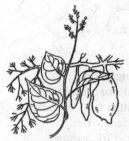

Fleeceflower root:
Bittersweet to the taste, warm in nature.
Tonic for the kidney and liver, good for ovulation, detoxifies, eases constipation. Used to treat hair loss due to iron deficiency caused by menstruation, sallow complexion etc.

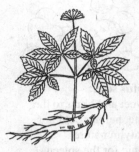

Ginseng root:
Sweet and slightly bitter to the taste, neither warm nor cold in nature. Boosts vital energy, spleen and lungs, promotes production of fluids and calms the mind. Good for cold limbs, fatigue and lethargy, poor appetite, weak constitution etc.

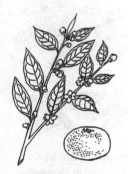

Tangerine peel:
Bitter and hot to the taste, warm in nature.
Regulates qi, strengthens the spleen, removes internal heat and phlegm. Good for qi stagnation in the spleen and stomach, poor appetite, cough with phlegm etc.

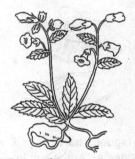

Rehmannia root:
Shengdi is bittersweet and cold in nature. Dispels heat, strengthens yin, promotes production of fluids, clots blood.
Shoudi is sweet and mildly warm. Good for the kidneys and blood, regulates menstruation and replenishes yin.

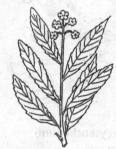

Loquat leaf:
Bitter to the taste, cooling in nature.
Dispels heat in the lung and treats cough, stops vomiting. Good for coughs due to heat in the lung, heavy breathing, thirst due to heat.

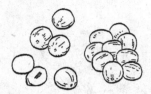

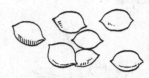

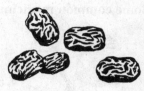

Lotus seed:
Sweet and bitter to the taste, neither cold nor heaty in nature.
Tonic for the spleen, stops diarrhoea, benefits the kidneys, calms the mind. Good for deficiency of the kidneys, prolonged diarrhoea, insomnia due to worry, incontinence and loss of sperm.

Gingko nut:
Bittersweet to the taste, neither cold nor heaty in nature, toxic.
Good for asthma, prevents parasites, controls urination. Used to treat coughs with phlegm, whitish discharge, incontinence, frequent urination.

Chinese date:
Sweet to the taste, warm in nature.
Replenishes qi, promotes blood and calms the mind, moderate medicinal properties. Good for weak spleen and stomach, deficiency of blood, insomnia, lethargy etc.

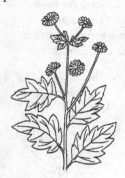

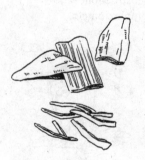

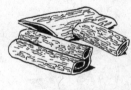

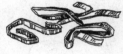

Chrysanthemum flower:
Bittersweet, cold in nature.
Dispels wind and heat, benefits the eyes and detoxifies. Used to treat colds due to external febrile factors, headaches, dizzy spells, infections.

Magnolia bark:
Bitter and hot, warm in nature.
Eliminates dampness and clears phlegm, treats stagnation of the qi. Good for discomfort of the spleen and stomach due to dampness, indigestion and stagnant qi; nausea, constipation, cough with excess phlegm.

Eucommia bark:
Sweet, warm in nature.
Tonic for the kidneys and liver, strengthens the muscles and bones, calms pregnancy. Good for joint aches due to failure of the liver and kidney, weak legs, unstable pregnancy, high blood pressure etc.

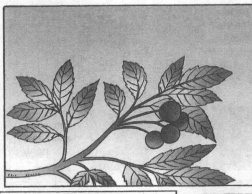

The Story of the Hawthorn Fruit

A sweet fruit, warm in nature. It aids digestion, dispels bruises, clears phlegm and clots blood.

Long ago, a stepmother tried to kill her stepson from her merchant husband's first marriage with his late wife during his absence.

I must remove this thorn in the flesh to let my own child inherit the money.

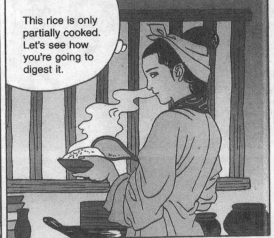

This rice is only partially cooked. Let's see how you're going to digest it.

If I complain about the rice, Stepmother will get angry. Let me just finish eating it.

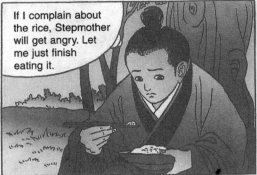

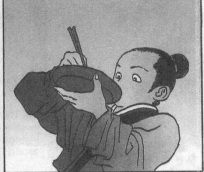

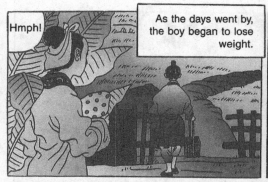

Hmph!

As the days went by, the boy began to lose weight.

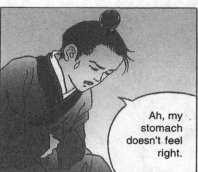

Ah, my stomach doesn't feel right.

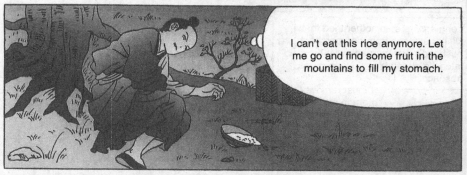

I can't eat this rice anymore. Let me go and find some fruit in the mountains to fill my stomach.

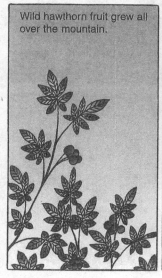

Wild hawthorn fruit grew all over the mountain.

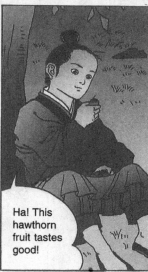

Ha! This hawthorn fruit tastes good!

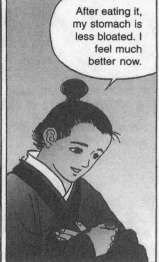

After eating it, my stomach is less bloated. I feel much better now.

58

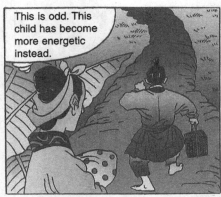

This is odd. This child has become more energetic instead.

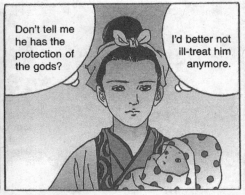

Don't tell me he has the protection of the gods?

I'd better not ill-treat him anymore.

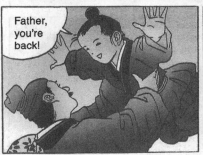

Father, you're back!

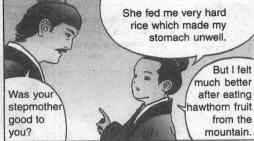

Was your stepmother good to you?

She fed me very hard rice which made my stomach unwell.

But I felt much better after eating hawthorn fruit from the mountain.

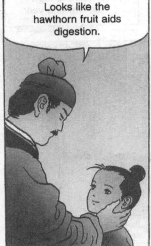

Looks like the hawthorn fruit aids digestion.

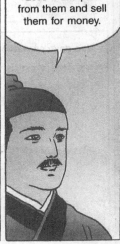

Let's make pills from them and sell them for money.

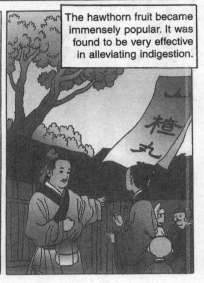

The hawthorn fruit became immensely popular. It was found to be very effective in alleviating indigestion.

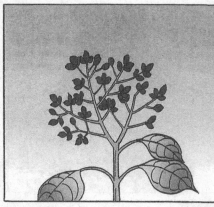

The Story of the Glossy Privet Fruit (*Nuzhenzi*)

A bittersweet fruit, neither cooling nor heaty in nature. It acts as a tonic for the liver and kidney, strengthens the back and knees, brightens the eyes, promotes black hair, alleviates swelling and relieves pain.

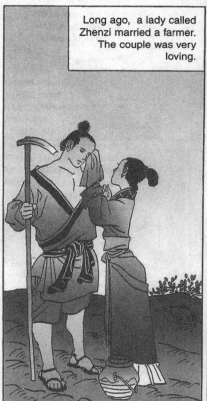

Long ago, a lady called Zhenzi married a farmer. The couple was very loving.

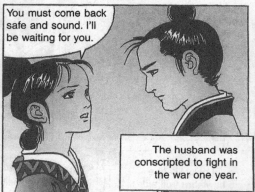

You must come back safe and sound. I'll be waiting for you.

The husband was conscripted to fight in the war one year.

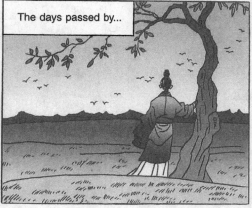

The days passed by...

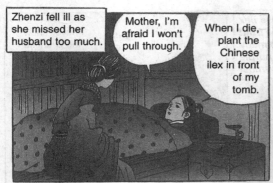

Zhenzi fell ill as she missed her husband too much.

Mother, I'm afraid I won't pull through.

When I die, plant the Chinese ilex in front of my tomb.

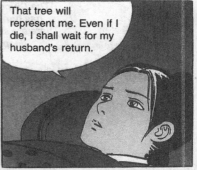

That tree will represent me. Even if I die, I shall wait for my husband's return.

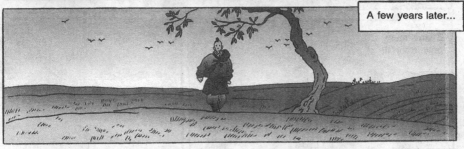

A few years later...

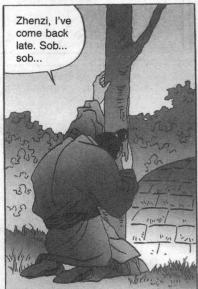

Zhenzi, I've come back late. Sob... sob...

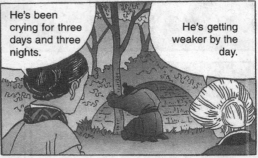

He's been crying for three days and three nights.

He's getting weaker by the day.

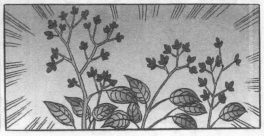

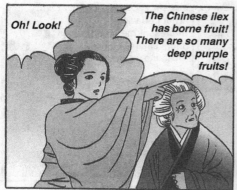

Oh! Look!

The Chinese ilex has borne fruit! There are so many deep purple fruits!

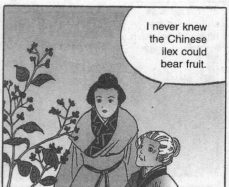

I never knew the Chinese ilex could bear fruit.

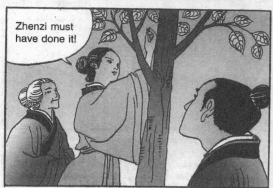

Zhenzi must have done it!

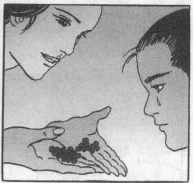

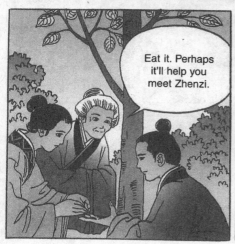

Eat it. Perhaps it'll help you meet Zhenzi.

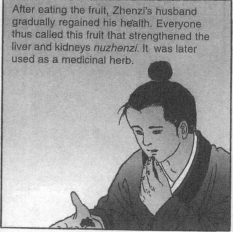

After eating the fruit, Zhenzi's husband gradually regained his health. Everyone thus called this fruit that strengthened the liver and kidneys *nuzhenzi*. It was later used as a medicinal herb.

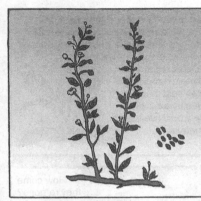

The Story of Wolfberries

Wolfberries: Sweet and neither cooling nor heaty in nature. A tonic for the liver and kidneys, promotes essence of life and brightens vision. Used to treat dizziness and ringing in the ears due to deficiency of yin in the kidneys and insufficient menstrual blood, worsening eyesight, aching back and knees etc.

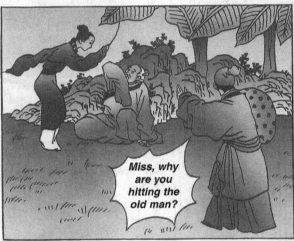

Miss, why are you hitting the old man?

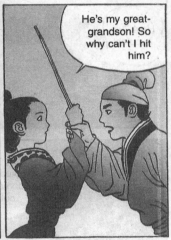

He's my great-grandson! So why can't I hit him?

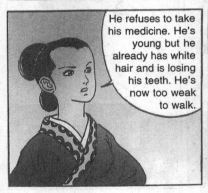

He refuses to take his medicine. He's young but he already has white hair and is losing his teeth. He's now too weak to walk.

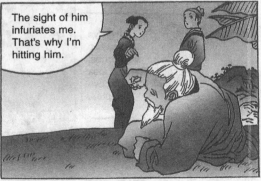

The sight of him infuriates me. That's why I'm hitting him.

63

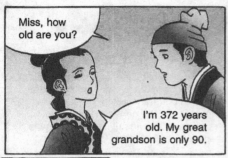

Miss, how old are you?

I'm 372 years old. My great grandson is only 90.

It turned out that this lady often took a particular medicinal herb called Essence of Heaven during springtime. In summer, it was known as wolfberries. In autumn, it was called earth bone and in winter, immortal's staff. It was said that if one ate it all-year round, he or she would live as long as heaven.

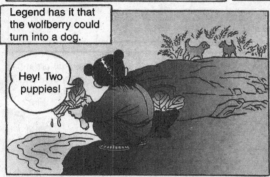

Legend has it that the wolfberry could turn into a dog.

Hey! Two puppies!

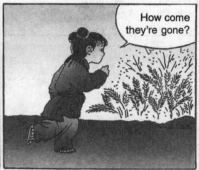

How come they're gone?

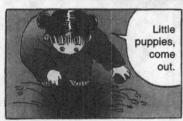

Little puppies, come out.

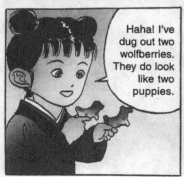

Haha! I've dug out two wolfberries. They do look like two puppies.

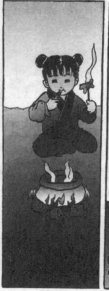

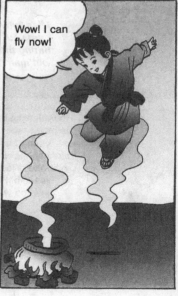

Wow! I can fly now!

Animal medicines

Animal medicines also include creepy crawlies like house lizards, centipedes, earthworms and silkworms, and aquatic animals like seahorses and seals.

Some examples of animal medicines

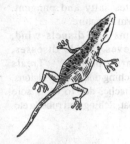

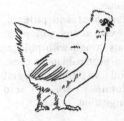

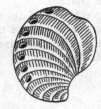

House lizard:
Tastes salty, cold in nature, mildly poisonous.
Expels wind, relieves pain caused by cold or dampness and soothes nerves. Used to treat paralysis due to stroke, numbness due to rheumatism, inflamed sores etc.

Black-bone chicken:
Tastes sweet, neither warm nor cold in nature.
Strengthens the kidneys, nourishes the qi and blood, dispels heat of deficiency type.

Abalone shell:
Tastes salty, cold in nature.
Detoxifies the liver and brightens the eyes, treats headaches and dizzy spells, blurred vision etc.

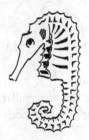

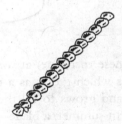

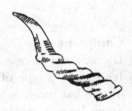

Seahorse:
Tastes sweet, warm in nature.
Strengthens the kidneys and improves virility, reduces swelling. Used to treat impotency, incontinence, deficiency of the kidneys, injuries due to a fall, difficulty in childbirth.

Centipede:
Tastes pungent, warm in nature, poisonous.
Expels wind and relieves febrile diseases, neutralises toxins, clears the channels and relieves pain.
Used to treat infantile convulsions, twitching, stroke, tetanus, poisonous snake bites, inflamed boils.

Antelope horn:
Tastes salty, cold in nature.
Subdues hyperactivity of the liver to calm endogenous wind, clears the liver and brightens the eyes. Used to treat high fever, fainting spells due to febrile diseases, bipolar disorder, headaches and dizzy spells etc.

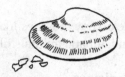
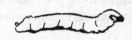

Leech:
Tastes salty and bitter. Neither cold nor warm in nature, poisonous.
Removes blood stasis, clears congestion and clears the channels. Treats bruises, injuries due to falls.

Clam shell:
Tastes bitter and salty, cold in nature.
Clears heat and phlegm, relieves aches and pain. Treats cough with phlegm due to heat, pain in the chest, blood in the phlegm, abdominal pain and acid regurgitation.

Silkworm:
Tastes salty and pungent. Warm in nature.
Calms and dispels wind, relieves febrile diseases, clears phlegm. Treats twitching due to convulsions, headaches due to wind, sore throat, itching and rubella etc.

Animal medicines such as bear gall, pilose antler, leopard bones and rhinoceros horn have caught the attention of animal activists. In their quest to lay hands on these animal parts for medicinal use, there has been poaching and killing of these animals. Also, often the methods used to obtain these medicines can be very cruel. That is why many Chinese physicians avoid using such animal parts in their prescriptions by substituting them with other medicines with similar properties.

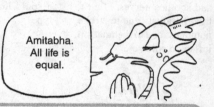

Amitabha. All life is equal.

Cordyceps

Is cordyceps (a type of Chinese medicine) a worm or a plant?
It's actually a type of fungus which grows as a parasite on the caterpillar of the bat moth in winter and grows to fill the caterpillar's entire body cavity, leaving only the skin. In summer, a blade-like leaf grows out. The fungus takes five to six years to reach maturity. As it resembles a worm, it is known as *dong chong xia cao* (literally meaning winter worm, summer plant). Cordyceps are mainly found in Sichuan, Qinghai, Guizhou and Yunnan. They are sweet-tasting and warm in nature. They nourish lungs and kidneys, stop bleeding, clear phlegm etc.

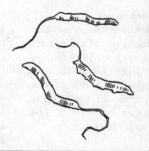

Minerals

Minerals are materials culled from nature which possess chemical properties. During the ancient times, minerals were also used in pill-making. In fact, minerals make up quite a substantial section in Chinese medicine.

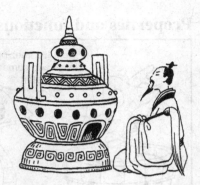

Some examples of minerals used in Chinese medicine

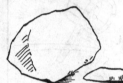

Gypsum: Tastes sweet and pungent. Cold in nature. Clears heat and expels fires, quenches thirst.

Realgar: Tastes pungent, warm in nature and poisonous.
Neutralizes poison, kills worms, especially effective in nullifying poisonous snake and insect bites. In ancient times, wine made with realgar was drunk during the Dragon Boat Festival.

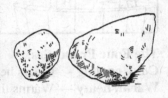

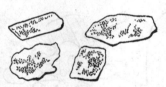

Mica: Tastes sweet. Neither warm nor cold in nature.
Nourishes the kidneys and relieves asthmatic symptoms, arrests bleeding and treats infection. Used to treat consumption of the lung and deficiency of the kidneys, asthma and asthmatic cough, dizzy spells, shock, inflamed sores.

Fossil fragments: Fossils left behind by prehistoric animals. Tastes bittersweet and neither warm nor cold in nature.
Calms nerves, arrests discharges. Used to treat an uneasy mind, insomnia due to anxiety, diarrhoea, seminal emission etc.

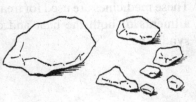

Properties and functions of Chinese medicine

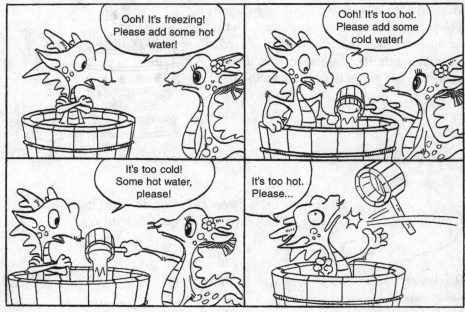

The Four Properties:

Cold, cooling — Clears heat, dispels fire, detoxifies
Warm, heaty — Warms the interior, dispels cold, promotes yang

Treatment for diseases of the heat syndrome uses medicines with cold and cooling properties. Conversely, medicines with warm and heaty properties are used to treat ailments of the cold syndrome. The principle of yin-yang balance is used here. Medicines which are not very strong are known as moderate medicines. These medicines are used for treating ailments of both the heat and cold syndrome.

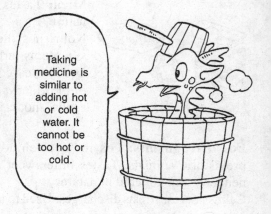

Taking medicine is similar to adding hot or cold water. It cannot be too hot or cold.

The Five Flavours:

Sour	Sweet	Bitter	Pungent	Salty
Arrests discharges, acts as an astringent.	Strengthens the body, balances the yin and yang, relieves pain.	Expels heat, reduces dampness, strengthens the yin, depresses fire.	Disperses internal heat, boosts circulation of the qi and blood.	Moistens, purgative effect.

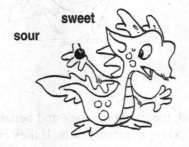

sweet

sour

Seldom does a particular medicine belong to one flavour solely. Generally, it may posses a few flavours to varying degrees. Therefore, many medicines possess more than one property.

Orientation and Location:

This refers to the location and orientation of the medicine in a person's body. It may be classified into two groups:

Ascending — promotes yang, to emit exterior heat of the exterior syndrome, dispels cold, induces vomiting.

Descending — reduces internal heat, purgative, diuretic, arrests inflammation.

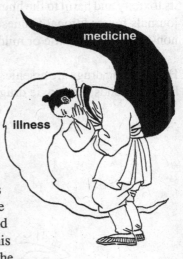

medicine

illness

An illness may affect a person in the upper part, lower part, exterior or interior. It may be identified as ascending, descending, exterior or interior in nature. Hence, treatment of the illness has to be in accordance with the nature of the illness. For example, a patient who vomits and coughs is suffering from an ailment that affects his upper body and is exterior in nature. Therefore, the medicine prescribed will be descending in nature.

Classification of medicines according to the meridians:

Illnesses often occur in different meridians and organs. Different drugs have different effects on each organ and meridian. The same drug that has effect on a particular disease may not be effective on another disease.

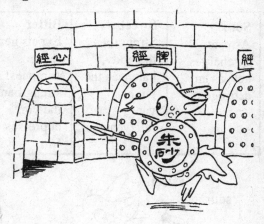

For example, Chinese ephedra is effective on diseases of the lung meridian but not the liver meridian; cinnabar works on the heart meridian but not the spleen meridian.

Toxicity

Medicines have two natures. On the one hand, they treat diseases and benefit the human body ; on the other hand, they are toxic to a certain extent. If they are not used correctly, they will cause harm to the human body.

In traditional Chinese medicine, the benefits of a medicine are enhanced while its toxicity and harm to the human body are reduced to the minimum. In medical journals for traditional Chinese medicine, every item will be labelled as toxic, non-toxic, highly toxic or mildly toxic.

Highly toxic drugs are arsenic, croton etc; mildly toxic drugs are pharbitis seed, bitter almonds; non-toxic drugs are poria and liquorice.

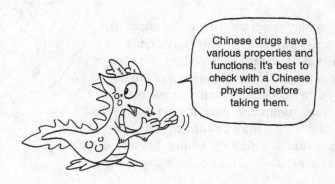

Chinese drugs have various properties and functions. It's best to check with a Chinese physician before taking them.

Making up a prescription

The combination of ingredients is known as a prescription. It combines the different properties of the various ingredients to enhance the effectiveness of the prescription. Alternatively, it also serves to moderate certain the side-effects of certain components used in the prescription and promote the effectiveness of the prescription.

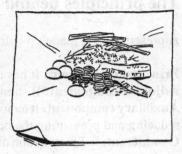

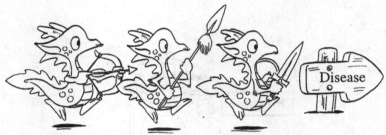

Taboos in preparing a prescription:
Some medicines cannot be mixed together as they may become toxic or decrease the effectiveness of the prescription. In traditional Chinese medicine, the taboos in preparing a prescription are known as the 18 Incompatible Medicaments and 19 Medicaments of Mutual Inhibition.

The 18 Incompatible Medicaments:

Aconite root (*wutou*) is incompatible with fritillary bulb, snakegourd fruit, pinellia tuber, *baijian*, bletilla tuber;
liquorice is incompatible with *gansui*, *dajian*, seaweed, genkwa flower;
lihui is incompatible with ginseng, *shashen*, *danshen*, *xuanshen*, *xixin*, peony root.

The 19 Medicaments of Mutual Inhibition:

Sulphur is inhibited by Chinese hackberry; silver is inhibited by arsenic; *langdu* root inhibits yellow lead; croton is inhibited by pharbitis seed; clove is inhibited by aromatic turmeric; nitre is inhibited by *jingsanling*; *chuanwu* and monkshood are inhibited by rhinoceros horn; ginseng is inhibited by *wulingzhi*; cinnamon is restrained by *shizhi*.

The principles behind a presciption

A prescription is made up with various principles in mind:

Principal component: It has the principal curative action.
Adjutant component: It strengthens the principal action.
Auxilliary component: It tempers the action of the principal ingredients, thereby reducing and preventing the occurrence of side effects.
Conductant: It directs action of the various components to the affected meridian or site.

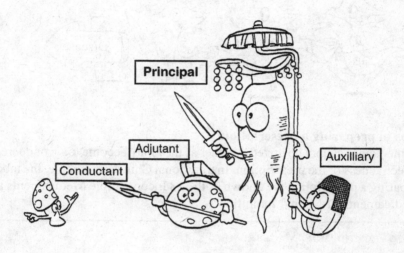

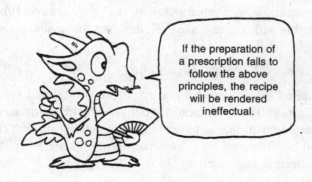

If the preparation of a prescription fails to follow the above principles, the recipe will be rendered ineffectual.

The Eight Principal Therapeutic Methods

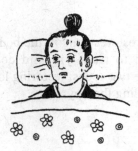

Perspiration
By inducing perspiration in a patient, the pathogenic factors are expelled from the body. This method is often used in the treatment of diseases caused by external pathogenic factors like colds and fevers.

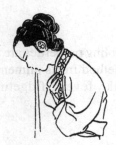

Emesis
Vomiting is induced in a patient. This method is used in the treatment of overeating, indigestion, food poisoning or congestion of phlegm.

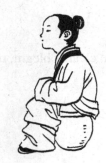

Diarrhoea
Laxatives are used to clear stagnation in the intestines and to relieve constipation or dysentery.

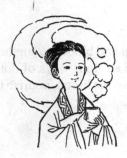

Soothing
Where inducement of perspiration and diarrhoea are not advisable, this method will be used in the treatment of diseases due to partial interior and exterior factors. Examples are a poor appetite, headaches and dizzy spells, thirst and bitterness in the mouth etc.

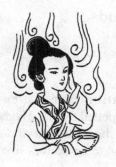

Warming therapy
It removes cold and restores yang in the body. It's primarily used to treat yin and cold syndromes. There are two types: restoring lost yang and cold-dispelling therapy.

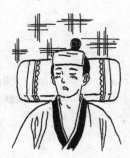

Heat reduction
Drugs with cold and cooling properties are used to reduce heat. This method treats ailments of the heat syndrome, like fevers, fidgetiness, fainting spells etc.

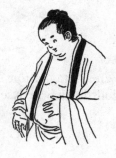

Relieve
Treats food stagnation, clears phlegm, reduces swelling etc.

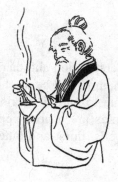

Tonics
Boosts the yin, yang, qi and blood; strengthens the constitution. There are four ways of doing it: nourish the qi, nourish the blood, nourish the yin and nourish the yang.

Methods of delivery in traditional Chinese medicine

Traditional Chinese medicine takes many forms. There are medicinal soups, pills, ointment and medicated wines.

Medicinal soup

This is the most common method for treating acute illnesses. The medicine is boiled as a soup, and the dregs drained away. It is absorbed into the body faster and results show faster.

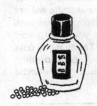

Pills

The medicine is ground into a powder and water or honey is added so that it can be rolled into balls. This method will take a longer time to show efficacy and is used over a longer period of time. It is ideal for chronic illness and prolonged weakness.

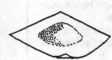

Powder

The medicine is ground into powder. It is taken with water for faster absorption or used in external applications. It is also applied in the throat and eyes.Ideal for acute illnesses.

Ointment

The medicine is decocted until it thickens into a jelly, which may either be consumed orally or applied externally. It is ideal for chronic illnesses or to replenish the body. External application is often done by pasting oiled paper or a plaster over the ointment to treat boils, corns or rheumatism.

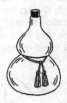

Medicated wine

The medicine is soaked in wine and the dregs are removed. It is quickly absorbed into the body and takes effect fast. Often used to treat rheumatic pains and injuries from falls or blows.

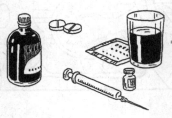

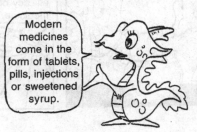

Modern medicines come in the form of tablets, pills, injections or sweetened syrup.

How to decoct medicine

Decocting medicine is not as easy as it seems. If it is not done properly, it will affect the effectiveness of the recipe.

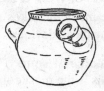

Pot

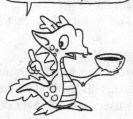

The best crockery to use are those made of ceramics as they will not have any chemical reaction with the drugs. As they conduct heat slowly, the medicine will not get burnt and stick to the bottom of the pot. Stainless steel and glass pots will also do. But you must avoid using bronze, aluminium and iron pots. These metal pots will have chemical reactions with the drugs and affect their effectiveness. They may even cause side-effects!

Washing the Pot

Pots used for decocting medicine should be washed thoroughly. The reasons are as follows:
• To prevent medicinal dregs from staying in the pot and interfering with the properties and effectiveness of the next brew.

• To prevent the dregs from settling at the bottom of the pot and becoming burnt.

Soaking the Medicinal Herbs

Before decocting the medicine, the herbs should be soaked in cold water for between 30 minutes to an hour. This is to enhance the efficacy of the herbs.

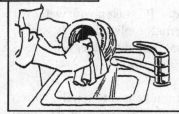

Some people will wash medicinal herbs as thoroughly as they would vegetables. Actually, this will make the herbs lose their qualities and affect the efficacy of the medicine.

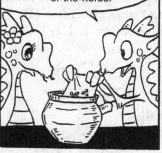

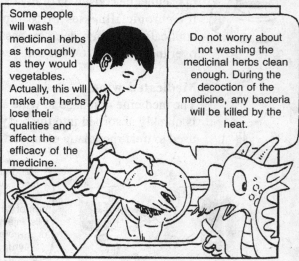

Do not worry about not washing the medicinal herbs clean enough. During the decoction of the medicine, any bacteria will be killed by the heat.

Amount of Water Added

Ideally, distilled water should be used to decoct Chinese medicine. However, drinking water will also suffice.

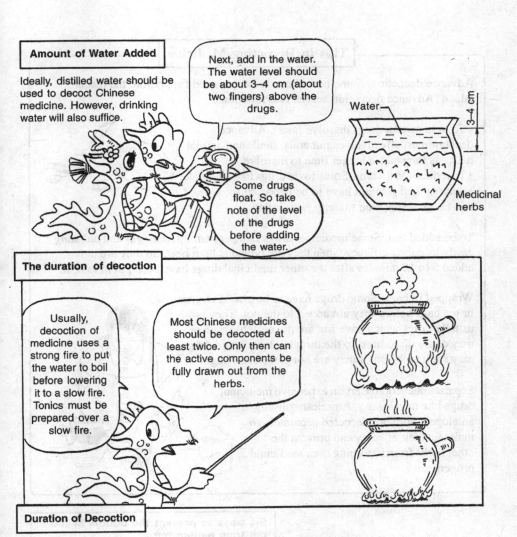

Next, add in the water. The water level should be about 3–4 cm (about two fingers) above the drugs.

Some drugs float. So take note of the level of the drugs before adding the water.

Water

3–4 cm

Medicinal herbs

The duration of decoction

Usually, decoction of medicine uses a strong fire to put the water to boil before lowering it to a slow fire. Tonics must be prepared over a slow fire.

Most Chinese medicines should be decocted at least twice. Only then can the active components be fully drawn out from the herbs.

Duration of Decoction

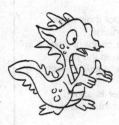

The amount of time spent to decoct the medicine depends on the type of medicine used and its medicinal purpose.

	First decoction	Second decoction
Medicine for general ailments	Bring to boil and cook for 30 minutes	Bring to boil and cook for 20 minutes
Medicine to dispel exterior heat syndrome	Bring to boil and cook for 8 – 10 minutes	Bring to boil and cook for 5 minutes
Nourishing medicine	Bring to boil and cook for 60 minutes	Bring to boil and cook for 30 minutes

Tips in Decocting Medicine

Advance decoction: Some herbs have to be decocted first before the rest are added. Advance decoction serves two functions:

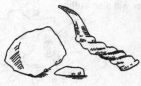

• To help certain drugs dissolve faster. Advance decoction usually involves minerals, shells and animal horns as they take a longer time to dissolve.
• To reduce the toxicity. Some toxic drugs like *chuanwu*, *shengfuzi* and *shanglu* have to be decocted for at least two hours before their toxicity is dispelled.

To be added last: Some medicinal drugs like peppermint. *danggui* and *dahuang* easily lose their efficacy when they are boiled at high heat. So they are only added 5 to 10 minutes after the other medicinal drugs have been put in to heat.

Wrapped in bags: Some drugs have to be placed in gauze or tea bags before they are added to the pot. They are usually drugs which have fur, are not easy to strain or may cause discomfort to the throat. Also, certain drugs may stick to the pot if they are not placed in a bag.

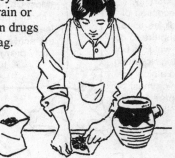

Separate decoction: Certain expensive medicinal drugs like the ginseng, American ginseng or antelope's horn are decocted separately to maintain their efficacy and prevent the other herbs from absorbing their medicinal properties.

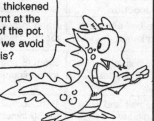

Often, we see the medicine thickened and burnt at the bottom of the pot. How do we avoid this?

Six ways to prevent the bottom of the pot from getting burnt:

1. Choose crockery that conducts heat evenly.
2. Clean the bottom of the pot thoroughly before decocting the medicine.
3. Place medicines that are sticky or fibrous in a bag before adding them to the pot.
4. Decoct the medicine over a low fire with the pot covered.
5. Make sure sufficient water is added.
6. Stir the mixture at regular intervals during decoction.

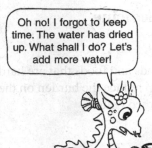

Taking the medicine

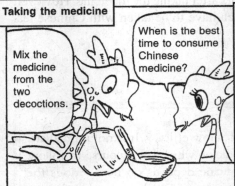

The times for taking the medicine depend on the nature of the medicine:

1. Consumption before a meal: Nourishing medicine.
2. Consumption after a meal: Medicine to dispel wind and dampness or medicine that is strong on the stomach.
3. Consumption on an empty stomach: Medicine to kill parasites and treat constipation.
4. Consumption before bedtime: Medicine to settle the mind and the heart.
5. Consumption without restricted timing: Medicine to treat exterior syndrome or acute illness.

Dosage:

Staggered consumption: Take one dosage once or twice a day. It is suitable for general illnesses. Chronic illnesses may require one dosage once every two days.

One-time consumption: Finish one dosage at one consumption. It is suitable for acute illnesses. Sufferers of serious illnesses may take two to three dosages a day.

Frequent consumption: The medicine is taken in small doses but more frequently. There is no fixed time to take it. It is usually the case for throat and oral cavity ailments.

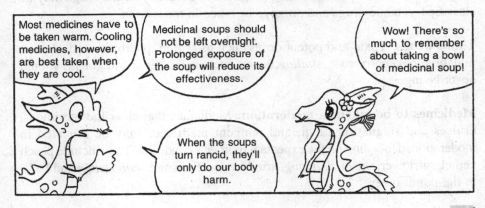

Things to note when taking Chinese medicine

Foods to avoid:
One should avoid taking cold and raw foods, oily foods and foods that are hard to digest when on Chinese medication. That will help reduce the burden on the digestive system and allow the medicine to be absorbed better.

At the same time, avoid garlic, onions and chilli.

Certain Chinese medicines should not be taken with Chinese tea. If you must have Chinese tea, drink it two to three hours after taking the medicine. However, there are certain Chinese medicines which have to be taken with Chinese tea. An example is the *chuanxiong* rhizome.

> **The course of Chinese medicine**
> Chinese medicine takes a longer time to show efficacy. It is not immediate. Chinese medicine is unlike western medicine which has a course to follow. In general, the course of Chinese medicine depends on how serious the disease is, the patient's response to the medication and many other factors. The course may be as short as a few days to as long as several years.

Medicines to be avoided during pregnancy
Certain Chinese medicines are harmful to foetuses and may induce miscarriage. They should never be taken during pregnancy. Generally, these drugs may be classified as taboo drugs and drugs to be taken in moderaton.

Taboo drugs: Toxic and potent drugs such as croton, pharbitis seed, *dajian*, mylabris, pokeberry root, *sanling*, leech, mercury, arsenic and *gansui* should never be ingested.

Medicines to be taken in moderation: Medicines that clear the meridians, bruises and stagnation of qi, and pungent medicines may be ingested in moderation, depending on the expectant mother's condition. They include peach kernel, safflower, *zhishi*, *dahuang*, dried ginger, cinnamon, *changshan* and Jack-in-the-pulpit tuber.

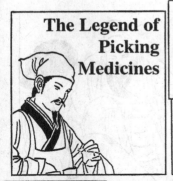

The Legend of Picking Medicines

We often see rows of little drawers behind the counter at a Chinese medical shop where the shop assistant will get the medicines from.

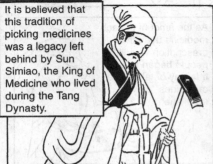

It is believed that this tradition of picking medicines was a legacy left behind by Sun Simiao, the King of Medicine who lived during the Tang Dynasty.

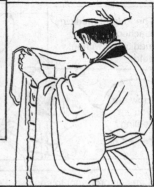

Sun Simiao often peddled his medical skill. Due to the many types of medicines he had to carry with him, he had an apron with many pockets sewn to store the drugs.

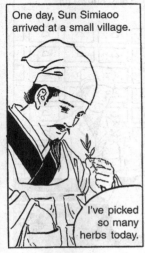

One day, Sun Simiaoo arrived at a small village.

I've picked so many herbs today.

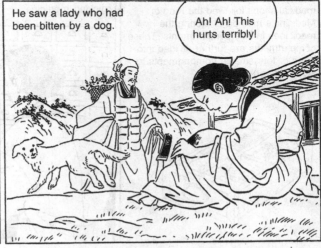

He saw a lady who had been bitten by a dog.

Ah! Ah! This hurts terribly!

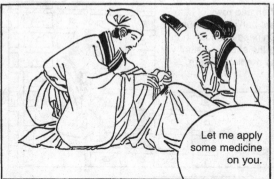

Let me apply some medicine on you.

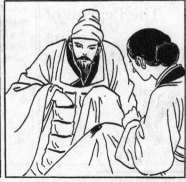

The King of Medicine reached for his medicines without delay.

How are you feeling?

The bleeding has stopped. It's also less painful now.

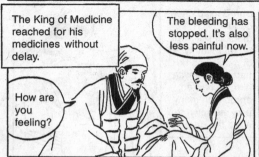

As the amount of each medicine used in a prescription was little, people began to call this way of taking the medicines 'picking medicine'.

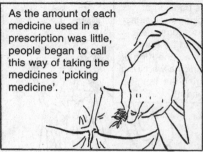

Later, in order not to confuse the wide variety of drugs, shopkeepers of medical shops followed the King of Medicine's method of storing the medicines in little compartments. These compartments are further divided into three or four smaller compartments to store different medicines.

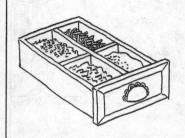

To this day, whenever one buys medicines from a medical shop, it is also known as picking medicine.

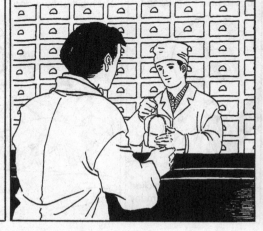

The Secret Prescription

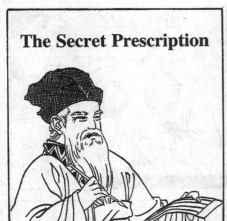

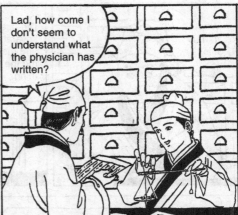

Lad, how come I don't seem to understand what the physician has written?

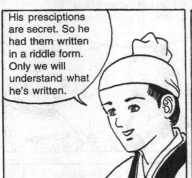

His presciptions are secret. So he had them written in a riddle form. Only we will understand what he's written.

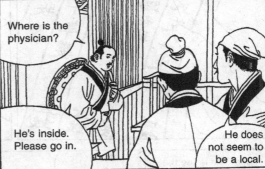

Where is the physician?

He's inside. Please go in.

He does not seem to be a local.

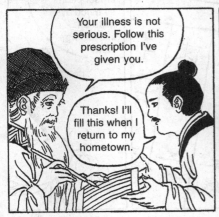

Your illness is not serious. Follow this prescription I've given you.

Thanks! I'll fill this when I return to my hometown.

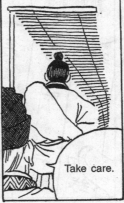

Take care.

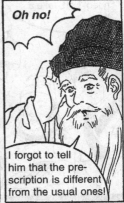

Oh no!

I forgot to tell him that the prescription is different from the usual ones!

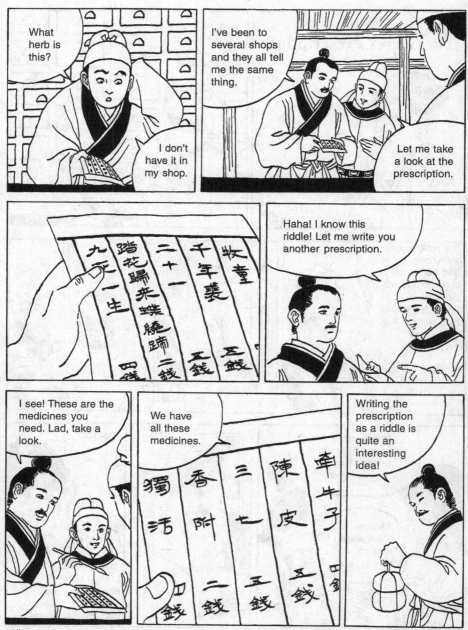

* Nine deaths and one life - duhuo (pubescent angelica root), Stepping on flowers are the butterflies - xiangfu, twenty-one - sanqi(notoginseng), Thousand-year attack - tangerine peel, shepherd boy - qianniuzi (pharbitis seed)

Table of commonly used Chinese medicines

For treatment of exterior syndrome (headaches, colds, etc):
Ephedra, saposhnikova root, fresh ginger, schizonepeta, *lanxiang* root, dahurian angelica root, peppermint, mulberry leaf, chrysanthemum, kudzuvine root, bugbane root.

Purgatives:
Rhubarb, honey, pharbitis seed, genkwa flower.

For expelling pathological heat:
Talc, abalone shell, aloe, selfheal spike.

For eliminating pathological heat from blood:
Bezoar, peony bark, gromwell root, *baimao* root, starwort root.

For eliminating heat-toxin:
honeysuckle flower, forsythia root, dandelion herb, oldenlandia.

For expelling heat:
Green bean, hyacinth seed, eupatorium.

For relieving rheumatic conditions:
Pubescent angelica root, acanthopanax bark, flowering-quince fruit, cocklebur fruit, *suanpanzi*.

For warming the interior:
Typhonium tuber, dried ginger, Chinese cinnamon, clove, fennel fruit.

For expelling dampness:
Poria, plaintain seed, wax-gourd peel, ricepaper-plant pith, loosestrife.

For expelling phlegm:
Jack-in-the-pulpit tuber, monkshood daughter root, milkwort root, fritillary bulb, seaweed, sea tangle.

Antitussives, expectorants and antiasthmatics:
Apricot kernel, balloonflower, gingko seed, loquat leaf, mulberry bark.

Table of commonly used Chinese medicines

For regulating the qi:
tangerine peel, flatsedge tuber, finger citron, eaglewood, cardamon, costus root.

For boosting blood circulation:
Chuanxiong rhizome, red sage root, peach kernel, *wenyujin* rhizome, turmeric root, sappan wood.

To arrest bleeding:
Notoginseng, agrimony, argyi wormwood leaf, burnet root.

To nourish the qi:
Ginseng, liquorice, Chinese date, *baishu*.

To nourish the blood:
Angelica root, fleeceflower root, mulberry fruit, mulberry mistletoe.

To nourish the yin:
Asparagus root, lily bulb, glossy privet fruit, solomonseal rhizome, wolfberry.

To nourish the yang:
Gecko, curculigo rhizome, dodder seed.

Sedatives/tranquilizers:
cinnabar, spiny jujube seed, silktree flower.

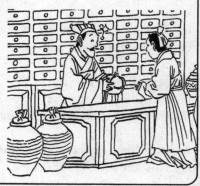

Method Two — Acupuncture and Moxibustion

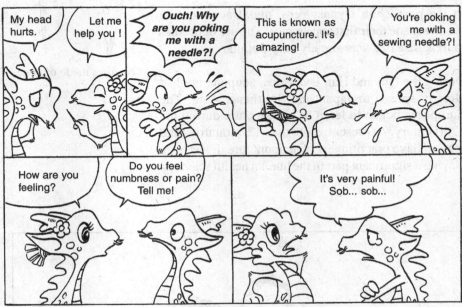

Isn't it amazing that a needle is able to relieve pain in the body?

Acupuncture and moxibusiton are remarkable features of techniques in traditional Chinese medicine. They are used in the treatment and prevention of many diseases. The effects are almost immediate and side-effects seldom arise.

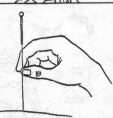

Acupuncture

Acupuncture and moxibustion are two different types of treatment. Both methods stimulate the acupoints on the body surface to bring about a harmony of the qi, blood, yin and yang in the afflicted body part.

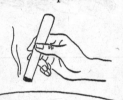

Moxibustion

The origins of acupuncture

These two methods of treatment can be traced back to the use of stone needles during the New Stone Age. At that time, they used needles of various shapes and sizes made from bones.

In the post-Zhou Dynasty era, metal acupuncture needles made their first appearance. The use of needles to treat diseases was already very popular.

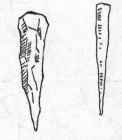

Needles made of bone

During the Qin and Han Dynasties, acupuncture had already spread to Japan and Southeast Asia. The Europeans began to learn of acupuncture during the 17th century. At present, more than 120 countries and regions have practitioners of acupuncture. It has been playing a significant part in the human health sciences.

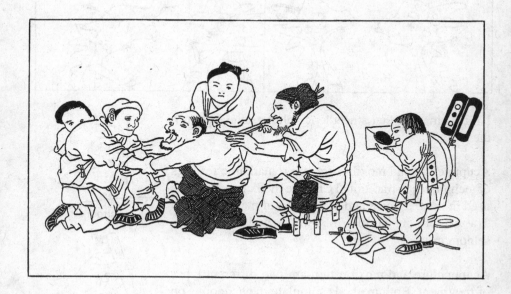

How acupuncture is carried out

Acupuncture involves the insertion of needles into the skin of a patient. Very fine needles made of metal or stainless steel are commonly used. They come in various lengths measuring from 15 milimetres to 100 milimetres. Their thicknesses also vary.

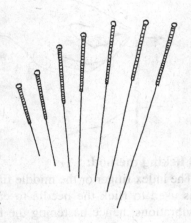

The acupuncturist will select the type of needles used based on the patient's state of health and physical condition. For example, in areas which are more fleshy and muscular, longer and thicker needles will be used. Shorter and finer needles are used for the chest and back areas.

After inserting the needle into the acupoint on the skin surface, he may move the needle in a variety of ways to exert varying degrees of stimulation on that acupoint. The patient will feel sore, numb and bloated in the spot where the needle has been inserted. This condition is known as 'getting the qi'. If such a condition is absent, it is probably due to the wrong acupoint being chosen and hence failure to treat the afflicted part.

Lift and thrust method:
When the needle has been inserted, the needle is lifted and thrusted into the skin surface or muscles.

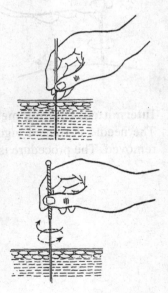

Rotating method:
When the needle is secured in the skin surface, the thumb, the index finger and the middle finger will then hold on to the needle and rotate it back and forth.

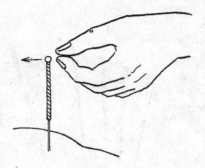

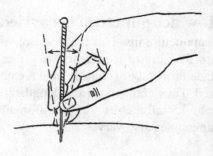

Flicking method:
The index finger or the middle finger is used to flick the needle to cause vibrations, hence hastening the flow of qi.

Rocking method:
Once the needle is inserted and secured, it is bent from side to side to allow the needle to make its impact greater.

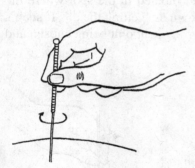

Intermittent rotating method:
The needle is rotated vigorously before the thumb and the index finger are removed. The procedure is repeated.

Ear-acupuncture therapy

The ear has reactive points with various diseases. That is why carrying out ear-acupunture on these points will effect treatment of diseases. Ear-acupuncture is used to treat a wide variety of diseases like various pains, phlegm, sensitivity, emotional upset, infectious diseases, chronic diseases etc. It may also be helpful in treating nicotine and other drug addictions as well as aiding weight loss etc.

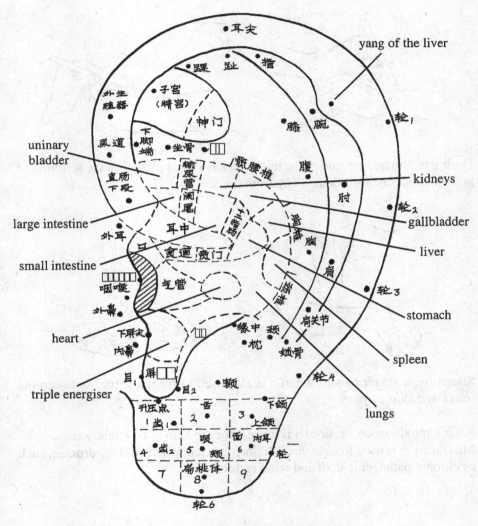

Diagram of acupoints in Ear-acupuncture.

Moxibustion

Moxibustion involves the use of lit moxa wool, a moxa stick or moxa cone to burn the acupoint, thereby regulating the qi and blood through the heat. Moxa is pungent to the taste and warm in nature. It therefore warms the collaterals and meridians and helps expel cold and dampness.

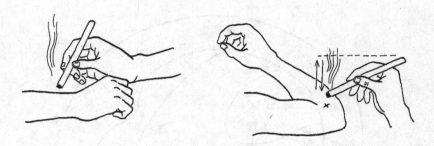

During treatment, one end of the moxa stick is lit and placed on the acupoint or held at about one milimetre away from the acupoint.

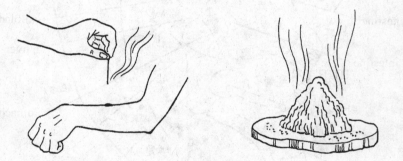

Sliced fresh ginger or sliced garlic is also used to form a barrier between the moxa and skin surface.

After a moxibustion session, it is normal for the skin to be slightly red. Moxibustion is used to treat yin, interior, deficiency and cold syndromes, such as chronic pathogenic cold and wind factors.

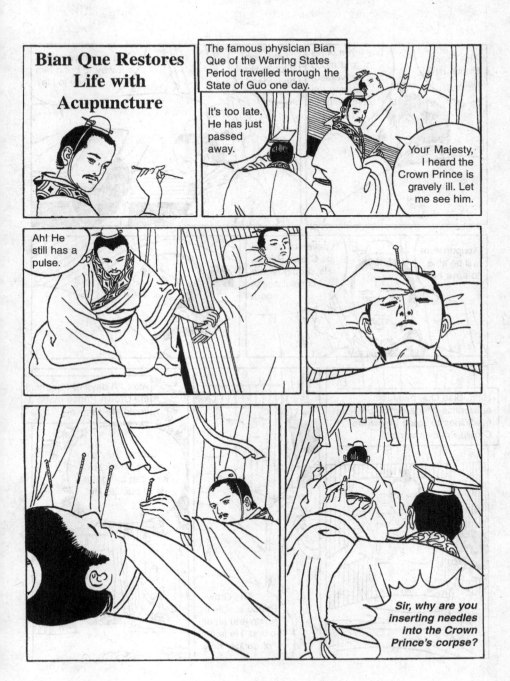

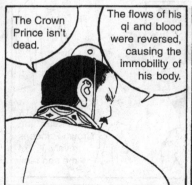

The Crown Prince isn't dead.

The flows of his qi and blood were reversed, causing the immobility of his body.

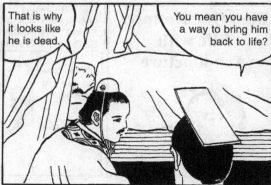

That is why it looks like he is dead.

You mean you have a way to bring him back to life?

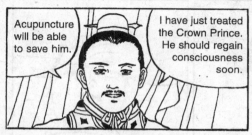

Acupuncture will be able to save him.

I have just treated the Crown Prince. He should regain consciousness soon.

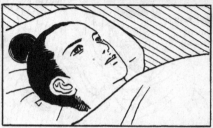

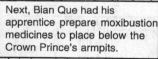

Next, Bian Que had his apprentice prepare moxibustion medicines to place below the Crown Prince's armpits.

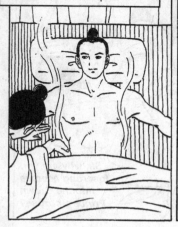

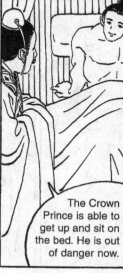

The Crown Prince is able to get up and sit on the bed. He is out of danger now.

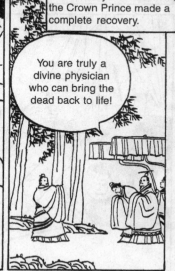

After 20 days of treatment, the Crown Prince made a complete recovery.

You are truly a divine physician who can bring the dead back to life!

Wang Weiyi Creates the Bronze Man

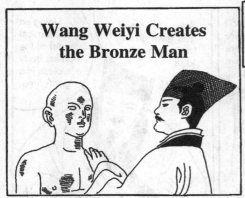

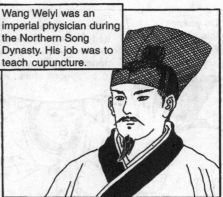

Wang Weiyi was an imperial physician during the Northern Song Dynasty. His job was to teach cupuncture.

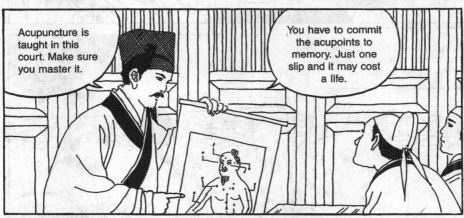

Acupuncture is taught in this court. Make sure you master it.

You have to commit the acupoints to memory. Just one slip and it may cost a life.

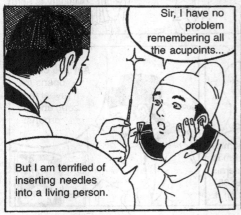

Sir, I have no problem remembering all the acupoints...

But I am terrified of inserting needles into a living person.

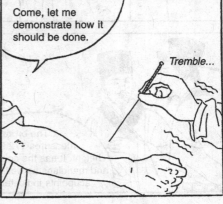

Come, let me demonstrate how it should be done.

Tremble...

95

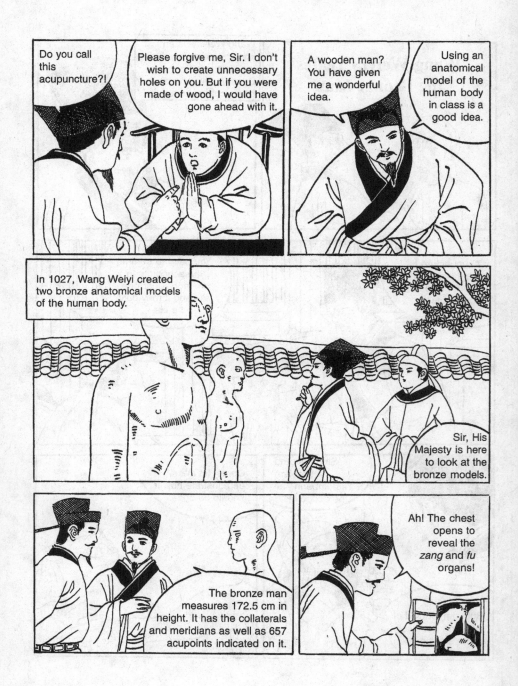

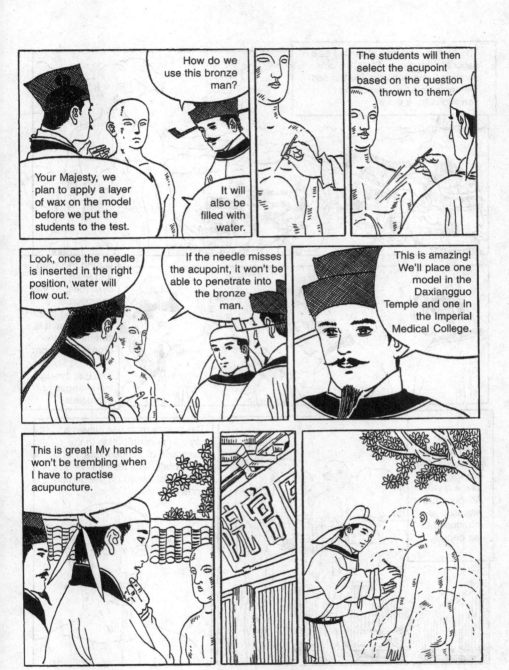

The bronze man was regarded as a national treasure. In 1128, the Jins invaded Song and even demanded the bronze man as one of the conditions for a truce.

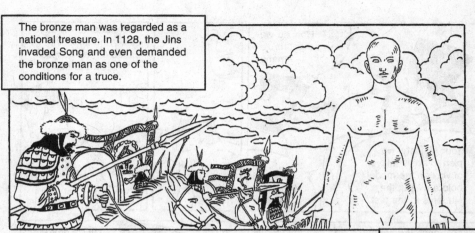

During the Yuan and Ming dynasties, further improvements were made to the bronze man. It is a shame that the bronze man from the Song Dynasty was lost through the changes of dynasties.

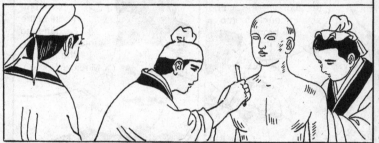

But during the Ming and Qing dynasties, the bronze man saw a revival. Acupuncture was thus re-introduced to the people.

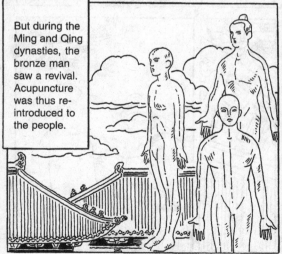

The bronze man has played a key role in contributing to the promotion of acupuncture. Incidentally, it is also the world's first model based on the human anatomy.

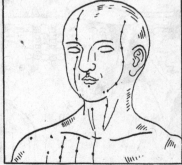

Method Three — Massotherapy

Massage pushes, presses, kneads or rubs the body to stimulate blood circulation, increase the skin's resistance level and regulate the nervous system.

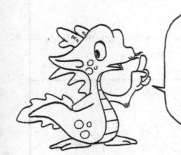

These days, the uses of massage have evol ved to include promoting good health and strengthening the physique. It is no longer limited to the treatment of diseases. Regular massage will relieve fatigue and perk one up!

Does massotherapy mean to 'push' and 'grasp'?

There are eight common types of massage. Pushing and grasping are just two types.

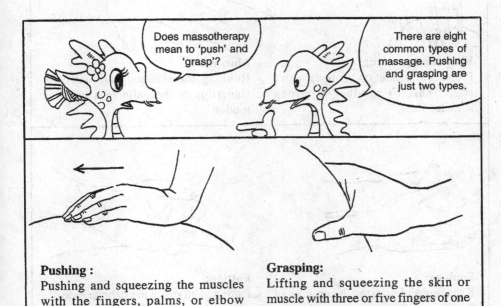

Pushing :
Pushing and squeezing the muscles with the fingers, palms, or elbow forward and backward.

Grasping:
Lifting and squeezing the skin or muscle with three or five fingers of one or both hands.

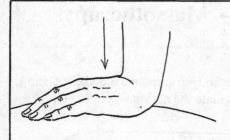

Pressing:
Pressing the acupoint or affected part with the thumb, palm or knuckle.

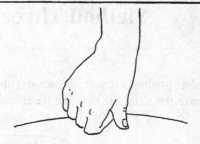

Tapping:
Tapping a point on the patient's body with the fingertips.

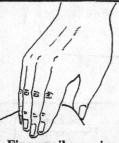

Fingernail-pressing:
Pressing at a point on the body with a finger-nail to produce a strong stimulation.

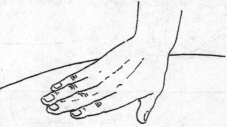

Massaging:
Rubbing the affected part with the fingertips or the palm in a circular motion.

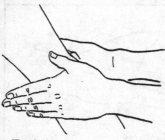

Foulage:
Kneading and pressing the muscles of the limbs with the palms.

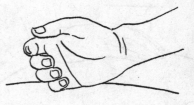

Patting:
Patting gently with the palm or side of the hand to cause relaxation.

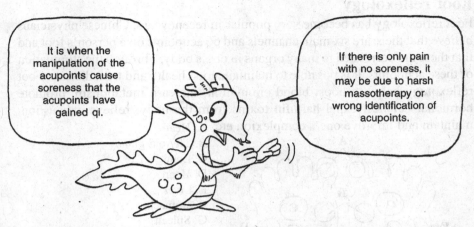

It is when the manipulation of the acupoints cause soreness that the acupoints have gained qi.

If there is only pain with no soreness, it may be due to harsh massotherapy or wrong identification of acupoints.

Massotherapy covers a broad spectrum of systems like the nervous system, muscular system, respiratory system, digestive system etc. It has been proven to be effective in treating ailments of these systems.

Cardiac Massage

We often watch on television how doctors will press on a patient's chest to try to return a regular heartbeat to the patient, thereby reviving him or her. This is also a technique used in massotherapy. During the Eastern Han Period, the famous physician Zhang Zhongjing introduced this method in *Synopsis of The Prescriptions of Golden Chamber*.

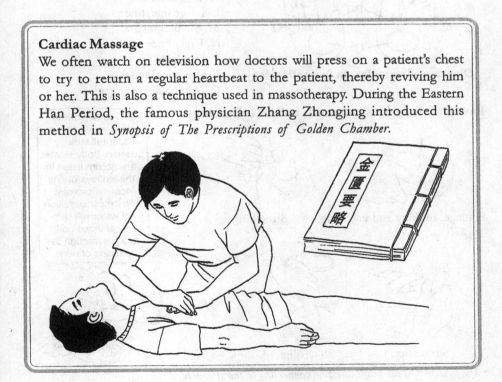

Foot reflexology

Foot reflexology has become very popular in recent years. Chinese physicians believe that there are six main channels and 66 acupoints on a person's foot and that these are correlated to many organs in one's body. Through the stimulation of these acupoints, it is possible to maintain good health and treat disease. Foot reflexology helps to boost blood circulation, increase metabolism, promote hormonal balance, expel harmful toxins from the body, relieve exhaustion, maintain and improve one's complexion etc.

A. Head
B. Thyroid gland
C. Lung
D. Heart
E. Liver
F. Stomach
G. Spleen
H. Pancreas
I. Right kidney
J. Left kidney
K. Duodenum*
L. Large intestine
M. Small intestine
N. Right knee
P. Left knee
P. Urinary bladder
Q. Reproductive organs

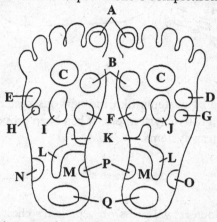

Diagram of acupoints in foot reflexology

There are four basic methods in foot reflexology:

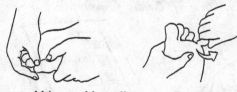

Foulage, rubbing and kneading   Stretching

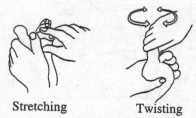

Stretching   Twisting

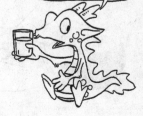

Do remember to drink water after a foot reflexology session. Body wastes are accumulated in the kidneys during foot reflexology. Hence consumption of water will help expel these body wastes through the passing of urine.

* The first part of the small intestine connecting to the stomach.

Other Methods in Foot Reflexology

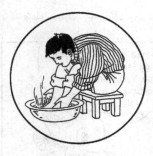

Washing the feet:
Traditional Chinese medicine believes that the act of washing feet also has massotherapeutic effects. The washing of feet is best done before bedtime. It is a simple method. Fill a basin with warm water and soak your feet in it. Rub your feet at the same time. This will not only clean the feet but also boost blood circulation, treat diseases and strengthen the constitution. You may also add marbles in the basin and step on the marbles.

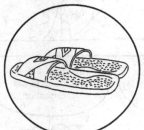

Wearing slippers with bumps:
Some slippers come with little bumps on them. Wearing these slippers also massages the feet.

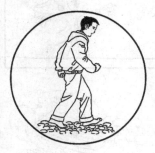

Walking on pebbles barefooted:
Walking on a pebbled path barefooted is like having foot reflexology and has therapeutic effects.

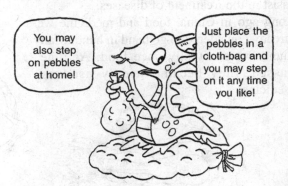

You may also step on pebbles at home!

Just place the pebbles in a cloth-bag and you may step on it any time you like!

Method Four — Diet Therapy

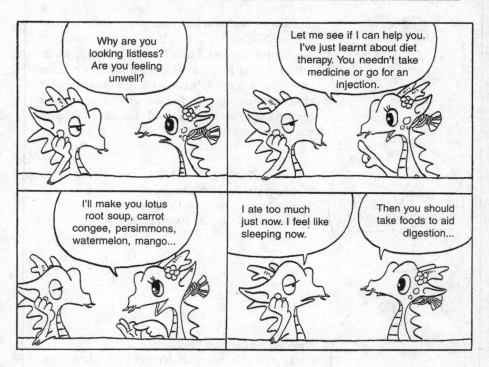

Diet therapy uses the food we eat daily to treat or assist in the treatment of diseases.

Long ago in China, food and medicine were already considered to go hand in hand. Many plants were actually once food. As time passed, they became widely used as medicines.

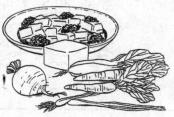

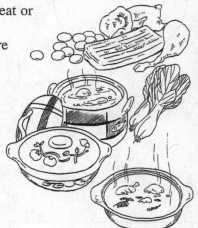

The famous physician Sun Simiao once said:

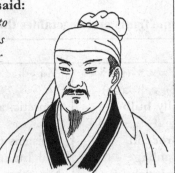

"To keep ourselves in good health, we have to depend on food. It is only in times of serious illness that medicines are prescribed. A poor knowledge of the right diet will not keep us healthy. A good physician ought to know the cause of a disease and find out where the afflicted part is. Treat the disease with diet therapy first. Prescribe medicine only if this fails."

Dieticians

In the Early Qin period, medical practitioners were already categorised into four groups: surgeons, physicians, dieticians and veterinarians. The dietician, in particular, would take care of the kings' and emperors' diets. He would plan the menu based on the season and the person's state of health to maintain the latter's good health and prevent disease.

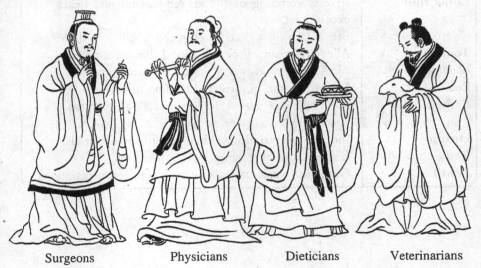

| Surgeons | Physicians | Dieticians | Veterinarians |

The relationship between diet and diseases

Some fruits and vegetables that prevent diseases:

Vegetables	
Caixin (flowering cabbage)	Aids digestion, promotes the metabolism.
Lily bulb	Diuretic, arrests bleeding, brings down swelling.
Leaf mustard	Improves vision.
Broccoli	Moistens the intestines, removes excess heat.
Cabbage	Benefits the kidneys.
Spinach	Nourishes the blood, removes excess heat and toxins, clears the intestines and stomach.
Bittergourd	Removes excess heat, nourishes the qi.
Towel gourd	Replenishes the blood, removes toxins and phlegm and relieves pain.
Cucumber	Diuretic, quenches thirst.
Winter melon	Removes excess heat, diuretic.
Fresh ginger	Disperses cold, prevents nausea, clears phlegm and toxins.
Lotus root	Arrests vomiting of blood, reduces fatigue, clears excess heat.
Carrot	Prevents infection, relieves facial swelling and toxins.
Tomato	Alleviates pain, disperses blood, lowers swelling.
Mushroom	Aids digestion, lowers blood pressure.
Pea	Nourishes the qi, arrests bleeding, diuretic.
French bean	Nourishes the blood, improves vision, prevents flaccidity of lower limbs.
Onion	Induces perspiration, aids digestion, treats colds.
Red pepper	Dispels cold and dampness, rejuvenates.
Lentil	Good for weak spleen and stomach, treats diarrhoea.

Fruits	
Mango	Treats coughs, nausea and dizziness.
Watermelon	Diuretic, relieves heat, treats inflammation of the kidneys.
Grape	Nourishes the blood, diuretic, treats liver diseases.
Pomelo	Aids digestion, neutralises toxins from alcohol.
Pear	Treats coughs and clears phlegm, quenches thirst, moistens the heart and lungs.
Sugar cane	Treats infection, nourishes the spleen, quenches thirst, clears toxins.
Loquat	Treats coughs and moistens the lungs.
Perssimon	Improves appetite, clears infection, treats coughs and moistens the lungs.
Longan	Nourishes the blood, sedative, improves appetite and nourishes the spleen.
Lychee	Quenches thirst, clears the mind.
Starfruit	Quenches thirst, clears heat, treats sore throats.
Papaya	Improves vision, clears heat, clears heat in the intestines, aids digestion.
Apple	Nourishes the heart and qi, promotes body fluid, quenches thirst.
Lemon	Helps in weight loss, aids digestion, clears the qi.
Banana	Quenches thirst, moistens the lungs and intestines, clears the blood vessel.
Guava	Diuretic, treats constipation.
Mandarin orange	Clears stagnation of qi, treats coughs and removes dampness.
Luohan fruit	Clears heat, treats coughs.
Pineapple	Quenches thirst, prevents heatstroke, brings down swellings and removes dampness.
Peach	Treats infection, clears blood clots, prevents constipation.

Others	
Red bean	Diuretic, treats flaccidity of lower limbs and water retention.
Green bean	Diuretic, clears heat.
Sesame	Nourishes the liver and kidneys; promotes blood.
Peanut	Arrests bleeding, improves the complexion, treats flaccidity of lower limbs.
Chestnut	Nourishes the kidneys.
Melon seed	Improves radiance, nourishes the qi.
Walnut	Improves complexion, promotes black hair, replenishes energy.
Olive	Good for hangovers, prevents coughs.
Sweet potato	Strengthens the spleen, stomach and kidneys.
Potato	Lowers blood pressure, treats gastric ulcers, asthma.
Corn	Strengthens one's body, nourishes one's brain, promotes bowel regularity.
Yam	Strengthens the intestines, treats diarrhoea.
Sunflower	Promotes blood, moistens the intestines.
Rose	Benefits qi and promotes blood, clears bruises and relieves pain.
Lily petals	Clears heat, sedative, prevents coughs and clears phlegm.
Chrysanthemum flower	Improves vision, clears heat, regulates blood pressure.
Beancurd	Clears the intestines and stomach, nourishes the qi.
Black moss	Nourishes the blood, promotes black hair.

The Five Flavours of food

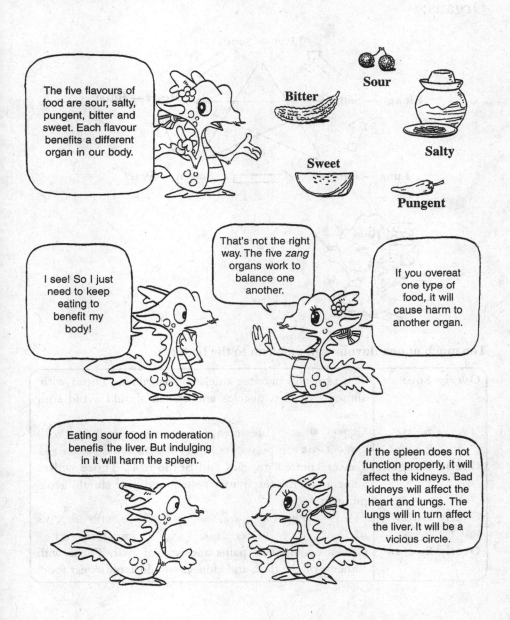

The five flavours of food are sour, salty, pungent, bitter and sweet. Each flavour benefits a different organ in our body.

Bitter

Sour

Salty

Sweet

Pungent

I see! So I just need to keep eating to benefit my body!

That's not the right way. The five *zang* organs work to balance one another.

If you overeat one type of food, it will cause harm to another organ.

Eating sour food in moderation benefis the liver. But indulging in it will harm the spleen.

If the spleen does not function properly, it will affect the kidneys. Bad kidneys will affect the heart and lungs. The lungs will in turn affect the liver. It will be a vicious circle.

The relationship between the Five Flavours and Five *Zang* Organs:

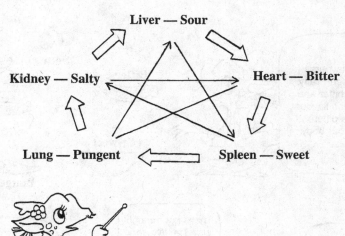

Liver — Sour

Kidney — Salty

Heart — Bitter

Lung — Pungent

Spleen — Sweet

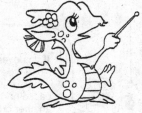

Too much of one flavour will do harm to the body:

Overly Sour	The skin will become thick and wrinkled. Those with ailments of the muscles and spleen should avoid sour food.
Overly Salty	Causes thirst, thickening of the blood. Those with ailments of the blood and heart should avoid salty food.
Overly Pungent	Causes knotted muscles and brittle nails. Those with ailments of the respiratory system and liver should avoid pungent food.
Overly Bitter	Causes withered skin and hair loss. Those with ailments of the bones and lungs should avoid bitter food.
Overly Sweet	Causes orthopaedic pains and loss of hair. Those with ailments of the flesh and kidneys should avoid sweet food.

The Four Properties of food

Food can be warm, heaty, cold or cooling.

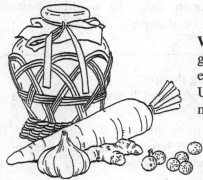

Warm and heaty foods: mutton, fresh ginger, garlic, carrot, longan, pepper, wine etc.

Uses: Builds the spleen, improves appetite, nourishes the kidneys, nourishes the body.

Cold and cooling foods: duck, crab, beancurd, spinach, bittergourd, pear, green bean etc.

Uses: Clears heatiness, brings down fire, detoxifies.

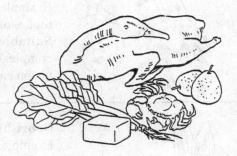

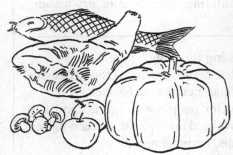

Foods that are neither warm nor cold: rice, soya bean, pork, carp, mushroom, apple, pumpkin etc.

Uses: Suitable for invalids and convalescents in general.

Four types of tonic

Tonics are usually foods prepared with medicinal properties. They are taken as part of the daily diet, having curative properties for someone who is ill and benefiting a healthy person. Before we take any tonic, we should understand our state of health in order to select one that will improve our health.

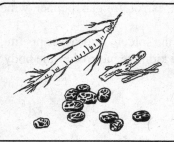

Nourishing the qi:
Examples: ginseng, Chinese dates, liquorice etc.
Suitable for people who are easily tired, short of breath, have poor appetite, perspire easily, down with a cold.

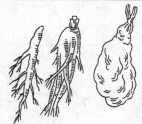

Nourishing the blood:
Examples: angelica, *shoudi*, fleeceflower root, wolfberry etc.
Suitable for people who have a pale complexion, get giddy spells and blurred vision easily, and suffer from insomnia.

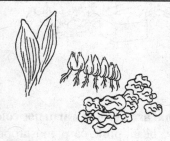

Nourishing the yin:
Examples: lily bulb, *shashen*, *zhimu*, white fungus etc.
Suitable for people with a weak constitution, insomnia due to stress, constipation, dizzy spells with ringing in the ears, dry mouth.

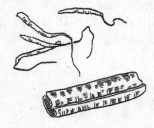

Nourishing the yang:
Examples: cordyceps, monkshood daughter root, Chinese cinnamon bark etc.
Suitable for people who are afraid of the cold, have cold limbs, weak and aching back and limbs, frequent urination.

Food taboos

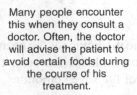

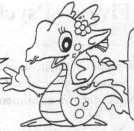

Many people encounter this when they consult a doctor. Often, the doctor will advise the patient to avoid certain foods during the course of his treatment.

Avoiding certain foods is based on the nature of the ailment to achieve a complete recovery and maintain one's health.

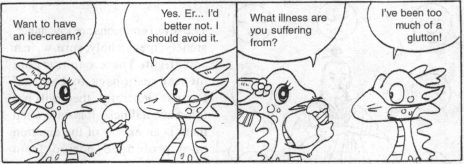

Want to have an ice-cream?

Yes. Er... I'd better not. I should avoid it.

What illness are you suffering from?

I've been too much of a glutton!

Foods to avoid during an illness

Ailment	Foods to avoid
High fever	Oily and spicy foods.
Insomnia	Strong tea, coffee.
Water retention	Salt.
Cold	Deep-fried foods, sweet foods, wine, chilli, white fungus.
Cough	Deep-fried or fatty foods, wine, pepper, prawn.
Diarrhoea	Fish, prawn, fried and deep-fried foods, fatty meat, fresh ginger, pepper.
Stroke	Salted meat and vegetables, fatty meat, coffee, strong tea.
Constipation	Wine, coffee, chilli, white fungus.
Asthma	Fatty meat, fish, prawn, crab, wine, soya bean, pumpkin, leaf mustard, carbonated drinks.
Diabetes	Sugar, sugar cane, fruit, sweet potato, starch, water chestnut, lotus, yam.
Kidney stones	Shellfish, asparagus, spinach, beancurd, lentil, persimmon.
High blood pressure	Organ meats, crab roe, egg yolk, chilli, wine, strong tea, coffee.
Jaundice	Fatty meat, deep-fried foods, chilli, wine, fish, prawn, crab.
Heart palpitations	Fatty meat, strong tea, coffee.

Method Five — Psychotherapy

There is a common saying: Ailments of the heart require medicine for the heart. This is in reference to psychological illnesses. Chinese physicians refer to ailments caused by psychological factors as ailments of the seven emotions.

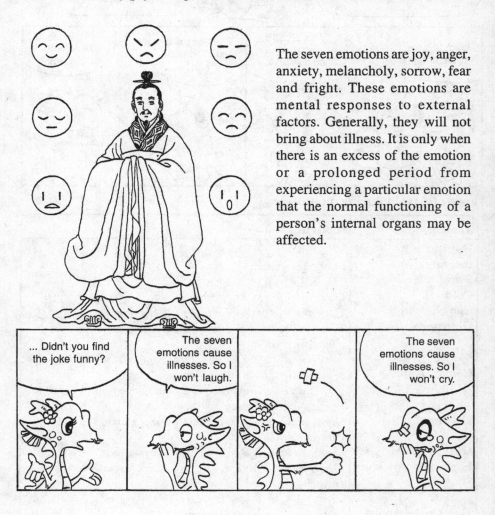

The seven emotions are joy, anger, anxiety, melancholy, sorrow, fear and fright. These emotions are mental responses to external factors. Generally, they will not bring about illness. It is only when there is an excess of the emotion or a prolonged period from experiencing a particular emotion that the normal functioning of a person's internal organs may be affected.

The Seven Emotions and their relationship with the Five *Zang* organs and Five Elements

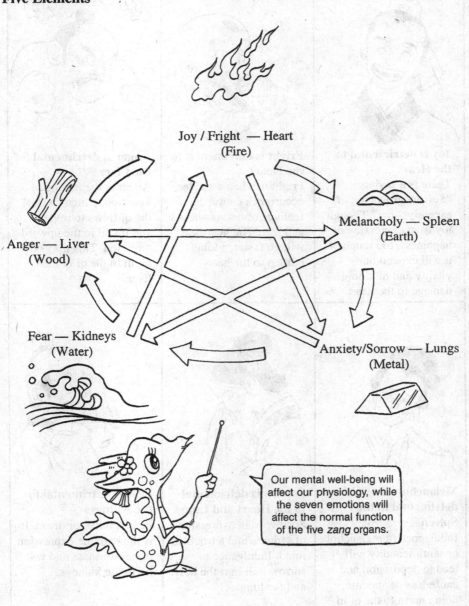

Joy / Fright — Heart
(Fire)

Melancholy — Spleen
(Earth)

Anger — Liver
(Wood)

Fear — Kidneys
(Water)

Anxiety/Sorrow — Lungs
(Metal)

Our mental well-being will affect our physiology, while the seven emotions will affect the normal function of the five *zang* organs.

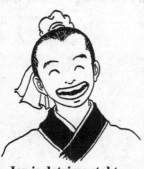

Joy is detrimental to the Heart
There is a saying: "Sorrow grows out of excessive joy." Though joy is an expression of happiness, too much of it will expend our vitality and qi, doing damage to the heart.

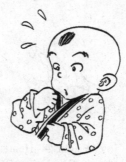

Fright is detrimental to the Heart
Fright is when a sudden occurrence causes feelings of nervousness and fear. The heartbeat will go faster, adding burden to the heart.

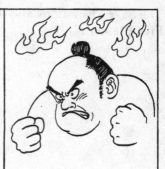

Anger is detrimental to the Liver
Anger is the feeling of agitation, which causes the qi flows to reverse and travel in the upward direction. This may do harm to the qi in the liver.

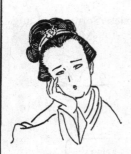

Melancholy is detrimental to the Spleen
Indulgence in melancholy or sentimentality will lead to depression and cause loss of appetite, doing harm to the qi in the spleen.

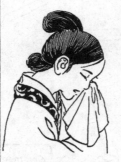

Sorrow is detrimental to the Heart and Lungs
Sorrow is an expression of sadness and a troubled mind. Indulgence in sorrow will hurt the heart and the lungs.

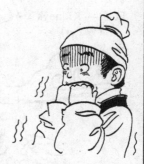

Fear is detrimental to the Kidneys
Fear is terror or dread. It is the extreme expression of nervousness and will harm the kidneys.

Overcoming or countering one emotion with another

As ailments of the heart require heart medicine, medicines will not do the job of treating the ailment. It is only by adjusting the emotions that the best treatment is achieved.

The seven emotions promote and restrain one another. One type of emotion will lead to another emotion:

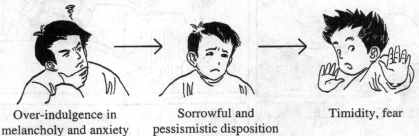

Over-indulgence in melancholy and anxiety

Sorrowful and pessismistic disposition

Timidity, fear

The method of overcoming one emotion with another involves curbing one emotion with another:

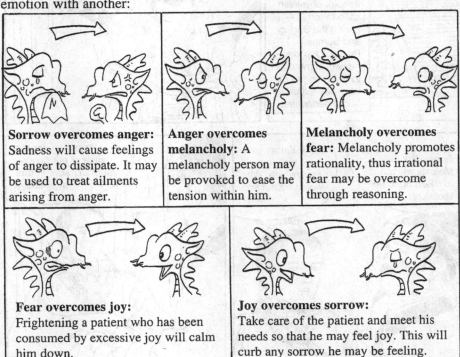

Sorrow overcomes anger: Sadness will cause feelings of anger to dissipate. It may be used to treat ailments arising from anger.

Anger overcomes melancholy: A melancholy person may be provoked to ease the tension within him.

Melancholy overcomes fear: Melancholy promotes rationality, thus irrational fear may be overcome through reasoning.

Fear overcomes joy: Frightening a patient who has been consumed by excessive joy will calm him down.

Joy overcomes sorrow: Take care of the patient and meet his needs so that he may feel joy. This will curb any sorrow he may be feeling.

The Famous Physician Who Was Cooked

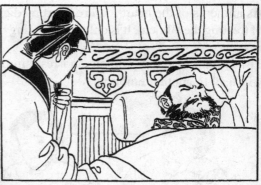

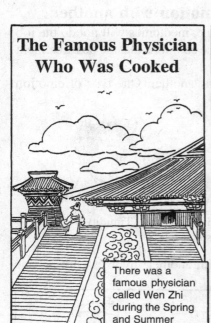

There was a famous physician called Wen Zhi during the Spring and Summer Period. One day, he was summoned to treat King of Qi who was suffering from headaches.

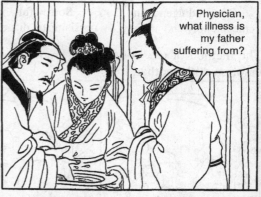

Physician, what illness is my father suffering from?

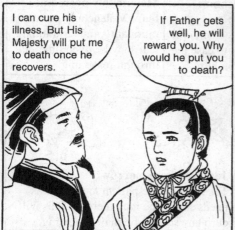

I can cure his illness. But His Majesty will put me to death once he recovers.

If Father gets well, he will reward you. Why would he put you to death?

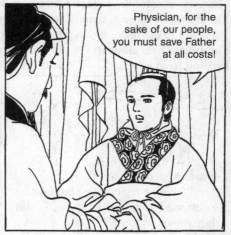

Physician, for the sake of our people, you must save Father at all costs!

118

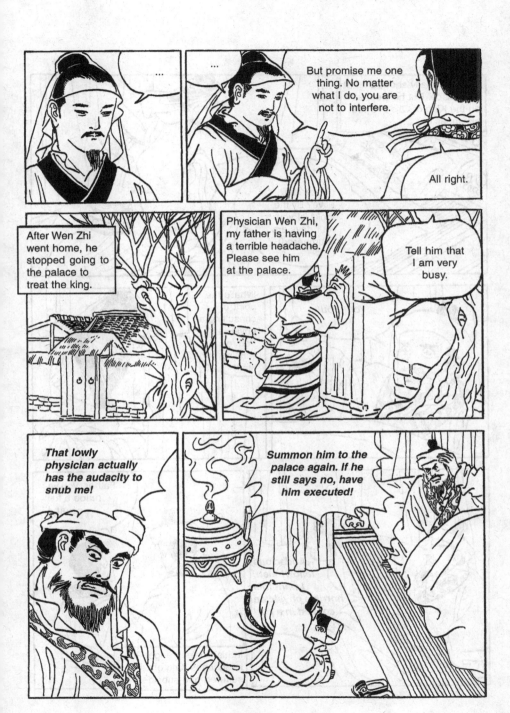

...

...

But promise me one thing. No matter what I do, you are not to interfere.

All right.

After Wen Zhi went home, he stopped going to the palace to treat the king.

Physician Wen Zhi, my father is having a terrible headache. Please see him at the palace.

Tell him that I am very busy.

That lowly physician actually has the audacity to snub me!

Summon him to the palace again. If he still says no, have him executed!

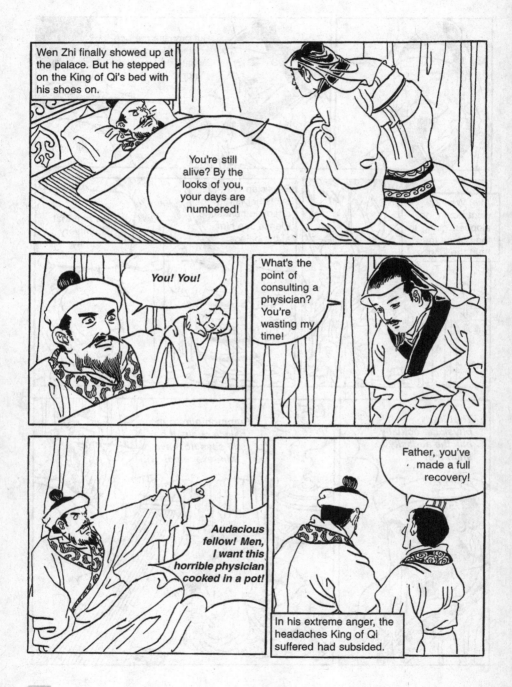

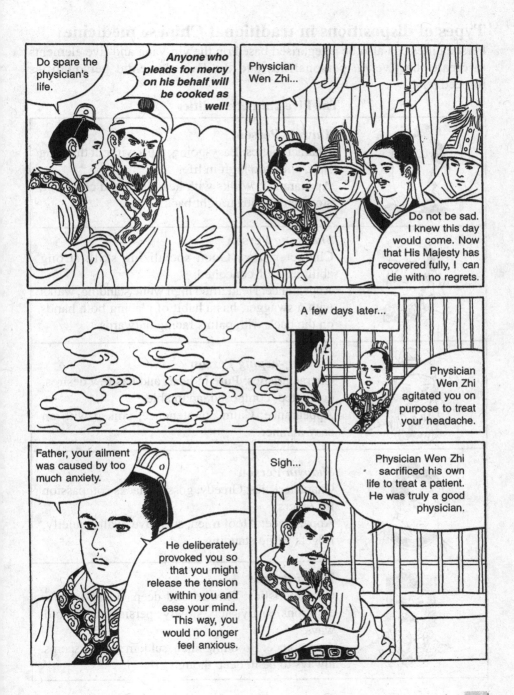

Types of dispositions in traditional Chinese medicine

Personalities can also be categorised based on the yin-yang and five elements to create the five *tai* personalities and the five elemental personalities respectively.

The Five *Tai* Personalities

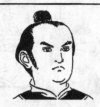

Taiyang Person
Characteristics: Easy-going, talks without thinking first, aims too high in life.
Appearance: Walks with head high and chest out, stomach in and straight back.

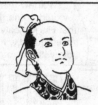

Shaoyang Person
Characteristics: Good socializing skill, strong abilities, self-conceited.
Appearance: Head lifted high while standing, walks with a swagger, has a habit of placing both hands on the back with palms facing outwards.

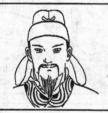

Yinyang-heping Person
Characteristics: Pure in heart and has few desires, contented, composed, adaptable.
Appearance: Calm countenance, poised with an easy manner.

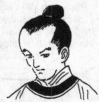

Shaoyin Person
Characteristics: Greedy, gossipy, lacks compassion for others.
Appearance: Aloof mien, secretive, walks quietly, fidgets while standing.

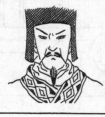

Taiyin Person
Characteristics: Shrewd and deep, doesn't show emotions easily, acts slowly, persists in his old ways.
Appearance: Brooding mien, seldom smiles, seems always to be in deep thought.

The Five Elemental Personalities

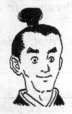

Fire Element

Characteristics: A quick worker, able to take stress, capable, generous and thinks little of money.

Appearance: Ruddy complexion, thin face, small head, small hands and feet.

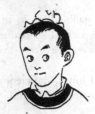

Metal Element

Characteristics: Both quiet and active, shrewd worker, honest.

Appearance: Pale complexion, square face, small head, small shoulders, small abdomen.

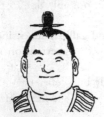

Earth Element

Characteristics: Trustworthy, keeps his emotions in check, helpful.

Appearance: Yellowish complexion, round face, big head, thick shoulder and back, large abdomen, small hands and feet.

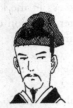

Wood Element

Charateristics: Talented and intelligent, introspective, melancholic, acts with motives.

Appearance: Pale complexion, long face and small head, broad shoulders and back, small hands and feet.

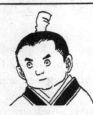

Water Element

Characteristics: Active, indecisive.

Appearance: Dark complexion, big head, small shoulders, large abdomen.

Diagnosis of illnesses through dream analysis

Our dreams are often tied to our emotional state, real-life experiences and encounters and our physical, among others. That is why dreams are able to reflect a person's state of health.

In *The Yellow Emperor's Medicine Classic — Miraculous Pivot*, dreams are classified in detail to diagnose illnesses.

Dream	State of Health
Fearful dream	Deficiency of qi in the heart and gallbladder, prolonged illness, excessive anxiety.
Angry dream	Stagnation of qi in the liver and gallbladder, as in hardening of the liver or the presence of gallstones.
Happy dream	Smooth flow of qi and blood, speedy recovery even if one should fall ill.
Sad dream	Deficiency of qi in the heart and lungs, deficiency of yin in the liver as with chronic liver disease and tuberculosis.
Melancholic dream	Imbalance in the liver and spleen, possibly due to poor food digestion and gastric ulcers.
Striving dream	Reverse flow of qi in the liver and gallbladder, rising of the yang in the liver as occurs with hypertension and poor food digestion.
Floating in dream	Excess in the upper part of body but deficiency in the lower part, like deficiency of the kidneys, excess phlegm, coronary heart disease.
Falling in dream	Deficiency in the upper part but excess in the lower part of the body. Often seen in water retention of the kidneys, deficiency of the yang in the heart.
Looking for food	Weak spleen and strong stomach, deficiency of yin in the stomach with pathogenic heat, gastric ulcers, intestinal parasites.
Looking for toilet	Often caused by stranguria (painful urination), inflammation of the intestines, poor digestion, diarrhoea.
Looking for drink	Mostly caused by excess yang and depletion of bodily fluids like due to high fever and dehydration.
Feeling cold in dream	Insufficient yang and heat, excess of yin and cold. Examples are deficiency of yang in the spleen and kidneys, interior cold syndrome.
Sleepwalking	Usually caused by stagnation of qi in the liver, distractions.

Traditional music therapy

With the growing acceptance of alternative treatments, music therapy has gained much attention. In fact, ancient physicians did considerable research on music therapy.

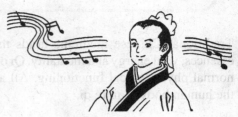

There are five notes in ancient Chinese music: *gong*, *shang*, *jiao*, *zhi*, *yu*. Chinese physicians matched each of these notes to a *zang* organ:

Gong (Do) — Spleen — Mediating nature
The note 'do' gives one a sense of calm and seriousness. It is used to treat someone who has been given a fright and is thus fidgety.

Shang (Re) — Lungs — Clearing nature
This clear and quiet note is used to treat someone suffering from anxiety and irritability.

Jiao (Mi) — Liver — Soothing nature
It creates a sense of softness, comfort and relaxation. It is used to dispel anger.

Zhi (Sol) — Heart —Invigorating nature
This note gives a sense of excitement and passion. It is used to treat someone with depression.

Yu (La) — Kidneys — Cooling and moistening nature
It is a melancholic note and acts as a sedative. It may be used to treat insomnia due to excessive joy or sorrow, heart palpitations etc.

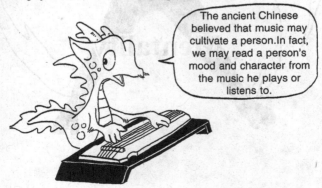

The ancient Chinese believed that music may cultivate a person. In fact, we may read a person's mood and character from the music he plays or listens to.

Method Six — *Qigong*

Traditional Chinese medicine holds that the human body consists of vital essences, vital energy and mentality. Qi or vital energy is the force that maintains normal physiological functioning. All activities of the *zang* and *fu* organs of the human body require qi.

There is congenital qi and acquired qi. Congenital qi begins in the mother's womb. It is the basic source of life. It is also called the Primordial Energy or Genuine Energy. Acquired qi is derived from air, food and other sources. Congenital qi depends on nourishment from acquired qi to carry out its functions.

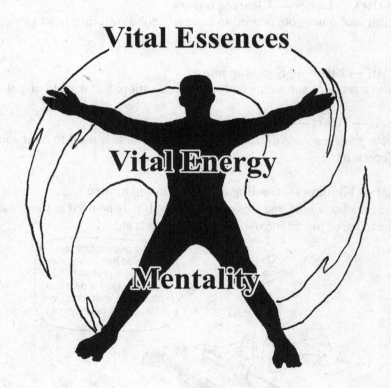

Vital Essences

Vital Energy

Mentality

When there is insufficient qi, the person will be listless, suffer general poor health and be susceptible to infectious diseases. By boosting the qi in the body, the functions of the *zang* and *fu* organs will be strengthened and the person will also become more energetic. But if the flow of qi is blocked or stagnates in the *zang* and *fu* organs, it will result in ailments of the body. That is why a smooth flow of qi is important for ensuring good health.

Deficiency of qi	Disruption in qi system
Stuttering speech	Easily agitated (depression of qi leading towards fiery disposition)
Feeling weak all over	Irritable and fidgety (depression of qi)
Pessimistic	Cough and shortness of breath (reversed flow of qi)
Gets tired easily	Bloated abdomen (stagnant qi)
Thin and weak breathing	Breathing difficulty (stagnant qi)
Panting and shortness of breath	Nausea (reversed flow of qi)

The practice of *qigong* will increase or boost vitality, thereby clearing the collaterals and meridians, replenishing qi in the blood, as well as harmonising yin and yang. It will treat diseases and boost the health of a healthy person.

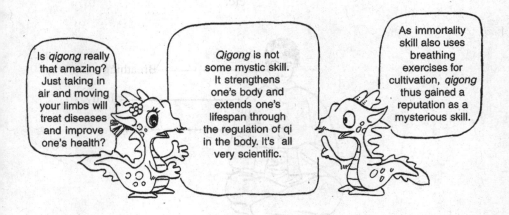

Is *qigong* really that amazing? Just taking in air and moving your limbs will treat diseases and improve one's health?

Qigong is not some mystic skill. It strengthens one's body and extends one's lifespan through the regulation of qi in the body. It's all very scientific.

As immortality skill also uses breathing exercises for cultivation, *qigong* thus gained a reputation as a mysterious skill.

At present, the US, Germany, Japan and other countries have set up research bodies on *qigong*. Many non-Chinese have also taken up *taijiquan* (*tai chi*) and meditation.

Qigong may be broadly grouped into two categories

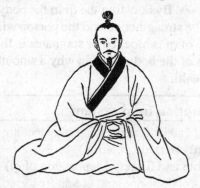

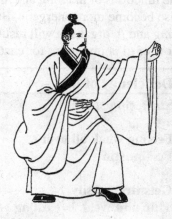

Internal exercise
Also known as static *qigong*, it emphasizes the training of the mental state. Methods include meditation, breathing exercises, relaxation etc.

External exercise
Also known as dynamic *qigong*. It promotes circulation of qi and blood through exercising one's muscles. Methods include gentle exercises like *taijiquan*, massage, conduction of qi etc.

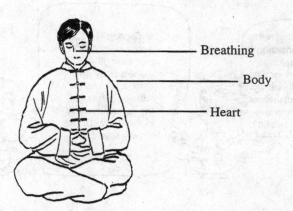

Breathing

Body

Heart

Whether it is dynamic *qigong* or static *qigong*, the emphasis lies in the regulation of the body, breathing and heart.

The effects of practising *qigong*

- A small abdomen and limbs that are warm to the touch.
- Slight perspiration.
- Increased salivation.
- The movement of the stomach and intestines becomes faster, resulting in a higher frequency of breaking wind.
- Increased appetite.
- Good sleep.
- A clear mind.
- The body feels light.

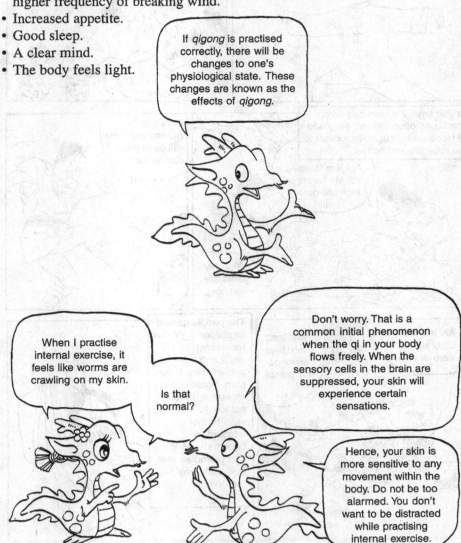

If *qigong* is practised correctly, there will be changes to one's physiological state. These changes are known as the effects of *qigong*.

When I practise internal exercise, it feels like worms are crawling on my skin.

Is that normal?

Don't worry. That is a common initial phenomenon when the qi in your body flows freely. When the sensory cells in the brain are suppressed, your skin will experience certain sensations.

Hence, your skin is more sensitive to any movement within the body. Do not be too alarmed. You don't want to be distracted while practising internal exercise.

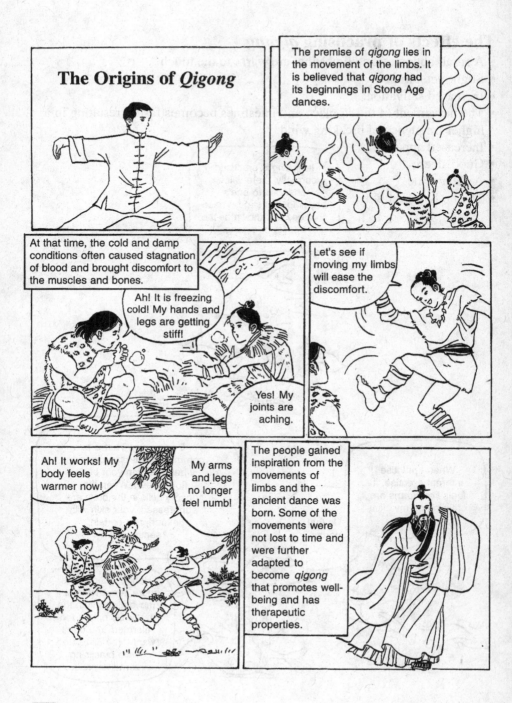

The Origins of *Qigong*

The premise of *qigong* lies in the movement of the limbs. It is believed that *qigong* had its beginnings in Stone Age dances.

At that time, the cold and damp conditions often caused stagnation of blood and brought discomfort to the muscles and bones.

Ah! It is freezing cold! My hands and legs are getting stiff!

Yes! My joints are aching.

Let's see if moving my limbs will ease the discomfort.

Ah! It works! My body feels warmer now!

My arms and legs no longer feel numb!

The people gained inspiration from the movements of limbs and the ancient dance was born. Some of the movements were not lost to time and were further adapted to become *qigong* that promotes well-being and has therapeutic properties.

Special Treatments

Other than the different methods of treatment introduced in the earlier pages, there are also special and highly unique therapeutic methods practised among the Chinese people.

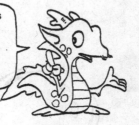

Examples are cupping, scraping and bloodletting.

Cupping

A small flame is placed inside a cup for a short while to heat it and expel any air within the cup. Using the principle of a vacuum, the cup is then sucked onto the skin surface to create local congestion in order to treat the ailment. This method is used in the treatment of rheumatism, expulsion of toxins and excess heat, to promote circulation of qi and blood, reduce swelling and relieve pain.

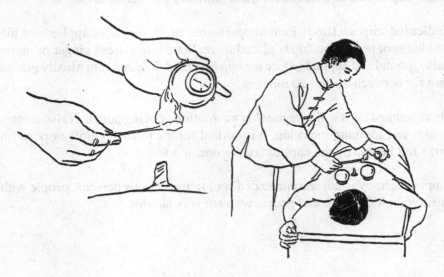

The cups made of glass used in cupping come in three sizes — large, medium and small. Their volumes range from 30 to 60 cubic centimetres. The glass around the cup rim is thicker to minimise the escape of air.

In the absence of glass cups, ceramic or other materials are also used. Some alternatives are teacups, wine glasses, small bowls or bamboo tubes.

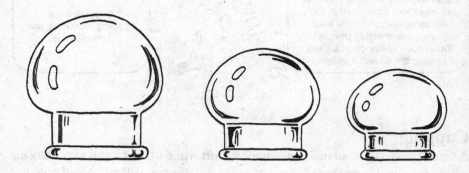

There are different methods used in cupping therapy:

Single-cup method: Suitable for the treatment of a smaller area.

Medicated-cup method: Pain suppressants or medicine is applied on the troubled spot before the cup is placed there. Sometimes, fresh ginger or garlic is also ground and applied before the cup is placed. The cups are usually placed there for between 10 and 20 minutes.

The vacuumed cups will give the skin a sensation of being pulled. It also creates a warm and soothing sensation. It is normal for the reddish purple or purplish marks left behind by the cups to last for one or a few days.

Cupping therapy is not recommended for highly nervous persons, people with sensitive or loose skin, and people who are very skinny.

Scraping

A copper coin or a small spoon dipped in oil or water is used to scrape the patient's chest, back, neck and other areas. Each area is scraped 20 times until purplish-red marks appear. It is used to treat dizzy spells, stuffy chest, bloated and painful abdomen, aching body etc.

In the past, the tools used in the scraping therapy were rather primitive. Copper coins, spoons and tile pieces were used, and very often, they caused bleeding and infections. Hence, it gave the impression of being primitive and unscientific. Nowadays, buffalo horns are used in scraping therapy. Buffalo horns are able to remove excess heat and expel toxins.They do not conduct heat and electricity. And the horns may be filed into various shapes and sizes to reach different parts of the body. In addition, the smooth texture of the horn is comfortable and will not hurt the skin.

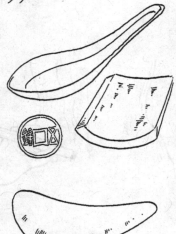

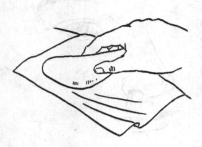

Before scraping, one should not have had a heavy meal or be starving. Scraping should only be done one hour after food and under the supervision of a trained physician. Patients who are suffering from blood diseases or bleed easily should avoid scraping therapy. A baby or young child undergoing scraping therapy should ideally have a sheet of cotton placed on the area to be scraped to avoid damaging the tender skin. Patients with skin problems should not go for scraping therapy.

Bloodletting

Needles or knives are used to pierce the acupoint or pulse to release a small amount of blood. It is ideal for patients suffering from heatstroke, high fever, poisonous bites or poisoning through ingestion etc.

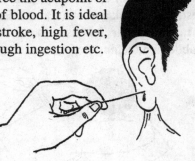

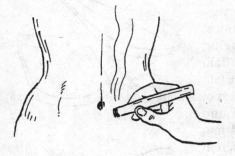

Umbilical cord therapy

Medicines, moxa sticks, heat, cupping and other therapies are used on the navel to treat various complaints, especially asthma, diarrhoea in young children, indigestion in young children, night terrors, irregular menstruation etc.

Nasal-insertion therapy

Medicines ground into powder are applied on a piece of cotton gauze which is then rolled into a stick. The cotton stick is then inserted into the nostril. It is used to treat nosebleeds, blocked nasal passages, toothaches, headaches, asthma etc.

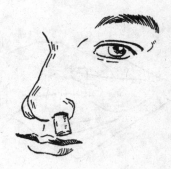

Medicinal pillows

Medicinal pillows are a type of treatment used in traditional Chinese medicine. Aromatic medicinal herbs that boost blood circulation and clear the channels are stir-baked before they are used as pillow filling. Sleeping on these medicinal pillows will help prevent diseases, fight ageing and prolong life.

The various types of medicinal pillows

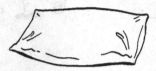

Cloth pillows:
Pillows made of cotton or gauze stuffed with herbs.

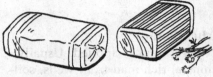

Wooden pillows:
The hollow part of the wooden pillow is stuffed with aromatic herbs. The wooden pillow is then wrapped in a piece of cotton cloth.

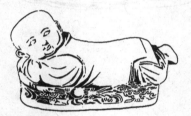

Stone pillows:
Stones and ceramics with medicinal properties are shaped into pillows.

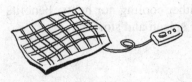

Electromagnetic pillows:
Electromagnetic gadgets are fixed to a traditional medicinal pillow to boost its effectiveness.

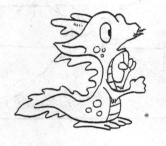

Whoa! So the hard wooden pillows our grandmothers used to sleep on had medicinal properties!

Dance therapy

Dance relaxes our muscles and boosts blood circulation. Not only does it strengthen the body, it can also be used to treat motor ailments like muscle cramps, stiff joints, etc. Ancient records reveal that dance was used to treat physical ailments.

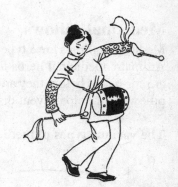

Mud therapy

Natural mud is applied. Usually, mineral-rich mud from wells, soil from farmland and yellow earth are used. Different types of mud possess different curative properties. For example, mud found in hot springs is warm, serving to boost blood circulation and free the meridians. Yellow earth, which is neither cooling nor heaty, benefits the spleen and stomach.

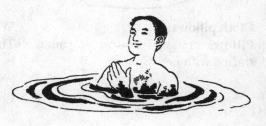

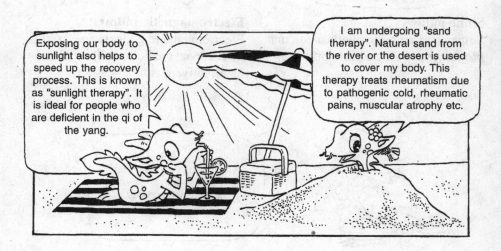

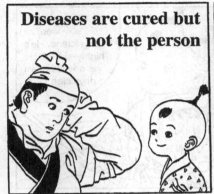

Diseases are cured but not the person

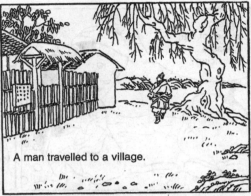

A man travelled to a village.

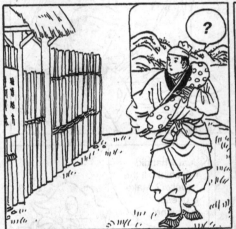

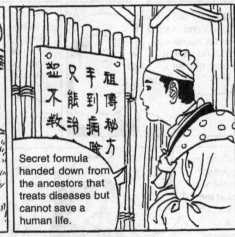

祖傳秘方 只能治到病除 翻不教

Secret formula handed down from the ancestors that treats diseases but cannot save a human life.

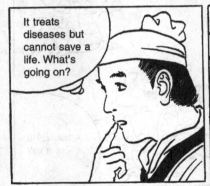

It treats diseases but cannot save a life. What's going on?

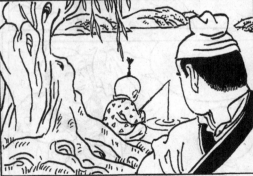

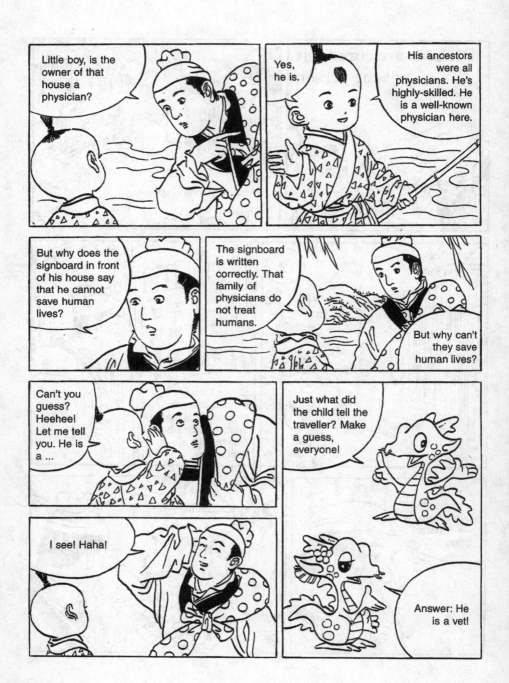

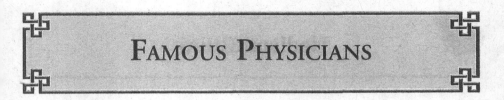

FAMOUS PHYSICIANS

Many top Chinese physicians have left their mark in the annals of Chinese history. These physicians not only possessed consummate medical skills, they also played an integral part in the development of Chinese medicine. More than just being gifted healers, they also possessed the highest moral integrity.

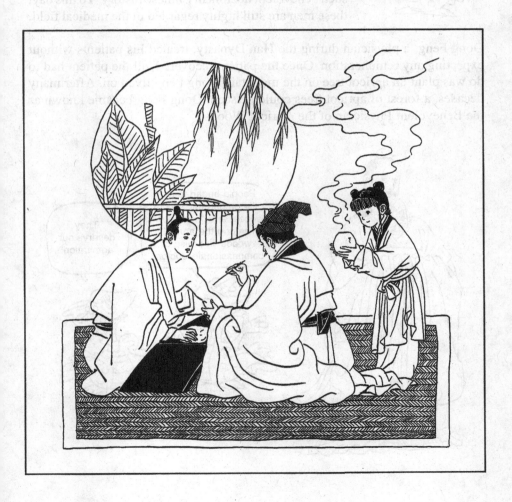

Medical Ethics

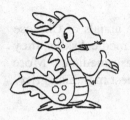

Medical ethics has been practised and advocated in China for a few thousand years. It advocates benevolence and compassion. Doctors do not just require excellent medical skills, they also have to be of an upright and moral character. There has been no lack of such benevolent doctors in Chinese history. To this day, these men are still highly regarded in the medical field.

Dong Feng, a physician during the Han Dynasty, treated his patients without expecting any remuneration. Once the patient recovered, all the patient had to do was plant an apricot tree on the mountain Dong Feng lived on. After many decades, a forest of apricot trees could be seen. Dong Feng became known as the Benevolent Physician of the Apricot Woods.

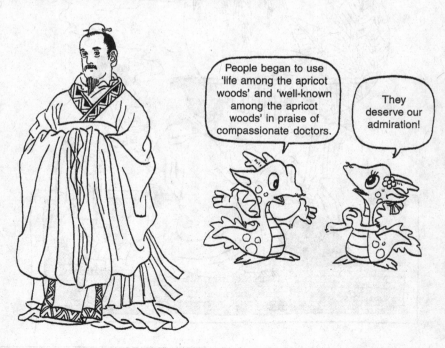

People began to use 'life among the apricot woods' and 'well-known among the apricot woods' in praise of compassionate doctors.

They deserve our admiration!

Bian Que

A famous physician during the Warring States Period, Bian Que introduced the Four Diagnoses of Illnesses — observation, ausculation and olfaction, interrogation and pulse taking.

Bian Que's birthname was Qin Yueren. He was the first physician to be recorded in Chinese history. Sima Qian of Western Han vividly narrated Bian Que's practice in *Records of the Historian — The Biography of Bian Que*.

In his youth, Bian Que worked in an inn. He later became an apprentice of Chang Sangjun to be trained in medicine. Legend has it that Chang Sangjun fed Bian Que some medicine which allowed him to see through walls so that he could look into his patients' *zang* and *fu* organs during consultation.

Bian Que was an all-rounder in the medical field, well-versed in internal medicine, surgery, gynaecology, paediatrics and others. As he travelled, he was able to adapt his skills to suit the culture and needs of the people in a particular place. In Handan, where the women were esteemed, he became a gynaecologist, while in Luoyang, where the elderly were held in high regard, he became an otolaryngologist (ear-nose-throat specialist). In Xianyang, he took up paediatric practice as the people there loved children.

Bian Que wrote the *Internal Classics of Bian Que* and *External Classics of Bian Que*, which have since been lost. The only surviving book is the *Classic on Medical Problems* written by Qin Yueren. This book expounds on the technique of pulse taking.

Bian Que's consummate medical skill was renowned. He travelled to many places to treat diseases among the people. Like the magpie or bird of joy, he brought good fortune to the people. Therefore he became known as Bian Que among the people though his birthname was Qin Yueren. However, his fame incurred the jealousy of imperial physician Li Xi of the State of Qin, who had him assassinated.

> **Bian Que's discourse on diseases:**
>
> *"When a disease is on the skin, use heat;*
> *if the disease is in the blood and pulse, treat it with acupuncture and moxibustion;*
> *if the disease occurs in the intestines and stomach, treat it with medicinal decoctions;*
> *but once the disease is in the bone marrow, not even a top physician will be able to do anything."*

Bian Que uses the Four Diagnoses on Marquis Qi Huan

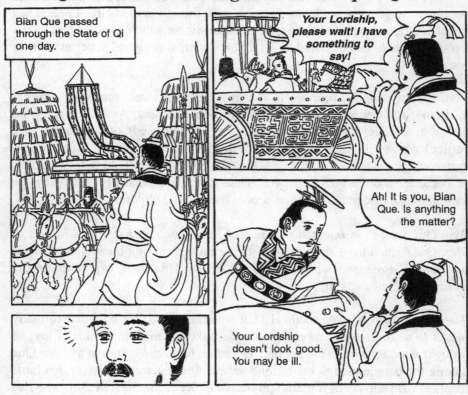

Bian Que passed through the State of Qi one day.

Your Lordship, please wait! I have something to say!

Ah! It is you, Bian Que. Is anything the matter?

Your Lordship doesn't look good. You may be ill.

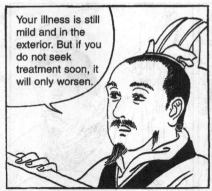

Your illness is still mild and in the exterior. But if you do not seek treatment soon, it will only worsen.

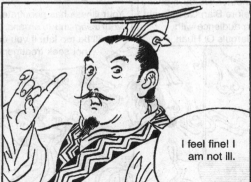

I feel fine! I am not ill.

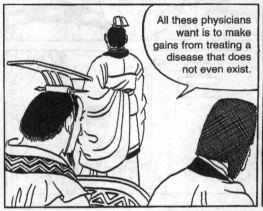

All these physicians want is to make gains from treating a disease that does not even exist.

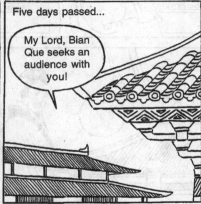

Five days passed...

My Lord, Bian Que seeks an audience with you!

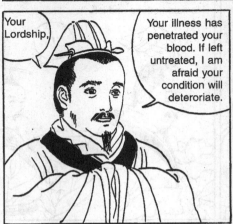

Your Lordship,

Your illness has penetrated your blood. If left untreated, I am afraid your condition will deteroriate.

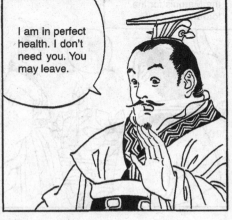

I am in perfect health. I don't need you. You may leave.

143

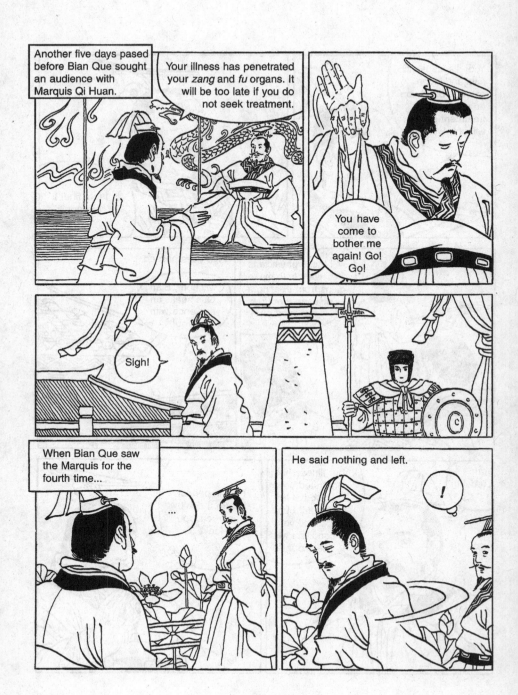

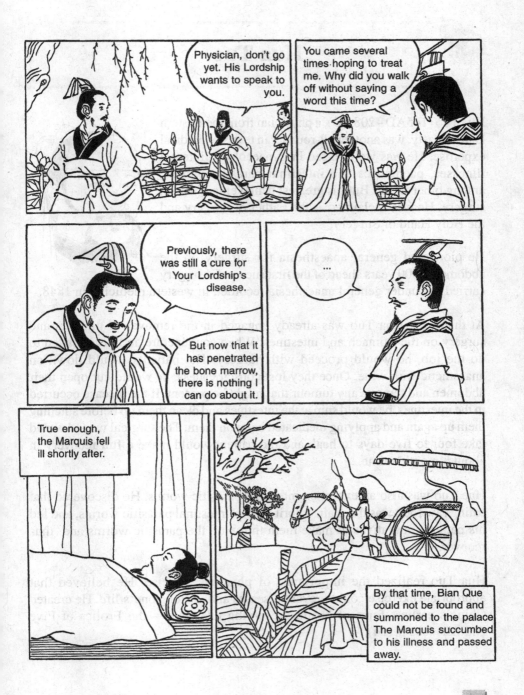

Hua Tuo

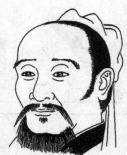

Hua Tuo (145AD - 208AD), a physician from the Eastern Han Dynasty, was another all-rounder in terms of medical expertise. He was well-versed in gynaecology, internal illnesses, paediatrics and intestinal parasitic worms, among other fields. But his greatest achievement was in surgery. He was acclaimed as the Father of Surgery and the Holy Hand of Surgery.

He pioneered general anaesthesia for surgery on the abdomen, 1600 years ahead of the first successful surgery carried out under general anaesthesia recorded in western medicine in 1848.

At that time, Hua Tuo was already engaged in the removal of tumours and surgery on the stomach and intestines. When acupuncture and drugs failed to do the job, he would proceed with surgery. His patients would down an anaesthetic with wine. Once they lost consciousness, he would cut open their abdomen and remove any tumour that might be present. If the disease occurred in the intestines, he would snip at the intestines and clean them up before stitching them up again and applying medicated balm on them. The surgical wound would take four to five days to heal, and the patient would make a full recovery in about a month's time.

Hua Tuo was also an expert on intestinal parasitic worms. He discovered that eating raw food was the main culprit behind intestinal parasitic worms, and fed his patients purgatives to make them throw up the parasitic worms and thus recover.

Hua Tuo realized the importance of physical exercise. He believed that appropriate exercise could prevent diseases and prolong one's life. He created China's earliest form of health-preserving exercise — the Frolics of Five Animals (see p.154).

146

He treated Cao Cao's severe headache and neutralised the poison in Guan Yu by scraping his bone. Unfortunately, Hua Tuo was later killed by Cao Cao. He complied his medical experience into a book known as the *Book of the Black Bag,* but it was lost after his death.

> **Hua Tuo:**
> *"Running water is never stale and a door-hinge never gets eaten by worms."*
>
> As running water is in constant movement, it never grows stale and smelly; a door-hinge turns every day, so it does not get eaten by worms. The human body needs adequate and suitable exercise. Exercise promotes food digestion, the flow of qi and blood and prevents diseases.

Hua Tuo Treats Severe Headaches

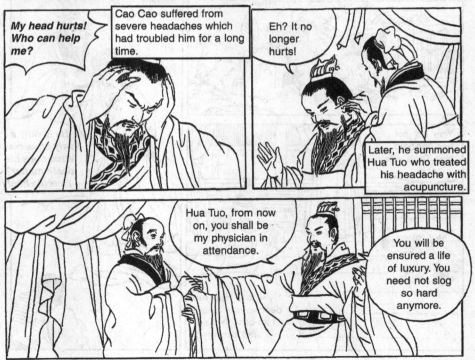

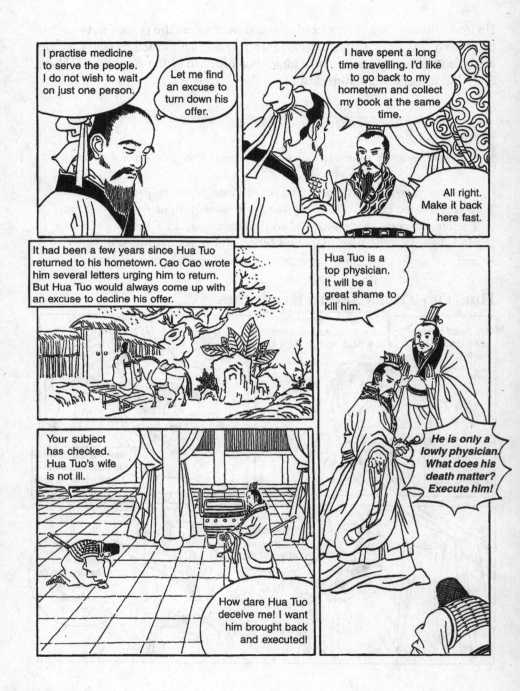

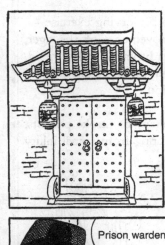

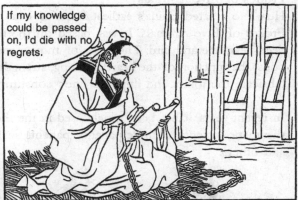

If my knowledge could be passed on, I'd die with no regrets.

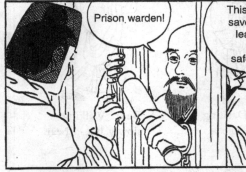

Prison warden!

This book will save lives. I'll leave it with you for safekeeping.

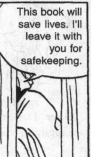

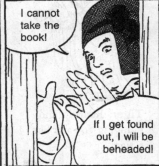

I cannot take the book!

If I get found out, I will be beheaded!

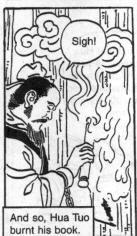

Sigh!

And so, Hua Tuo burnt his book.

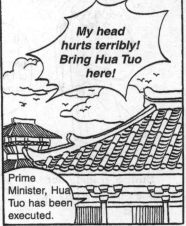

My head hurts terribly! Bring Hua Tuo here!

Prime Minister, Hua Tuo has been executed.

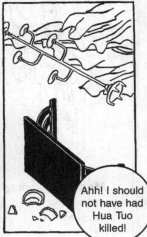

Ahh! I should not have had Hua Tuo killed!

Frolics of Five Animals

Hua Tuo created China's earliest form of health-preserving exercise — Frolics of Five Animals. It was based on the movements of the tiger, deer, bear, ape and bird. The series of movements promote a clear mind, boost the function of the heart and lung, strengthen the back and kidneys, lubricate the joints and improve one's constitution.

In recent years, it has been widely used in the therapy of stroke patients, rheumatic patients, arthritic patients, patients suffering from spinal injury and others.

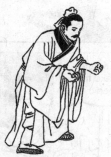

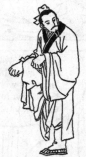

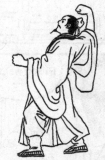

Tiger: Roaring and plunging foward like a tiger.

Deer: Dashing happily like a deer.

Bear: Walking slowly like a bear.

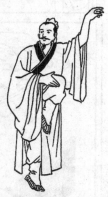

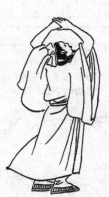

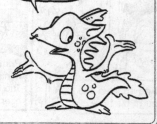

It is said that Hua Tuo's disciple who practised the Frolics of Five Animals lived to over 100 years of age!

Monkey: Jumping around like a monkey.

Bird: Spreading out one's hands to fly like a bird.

Zhang Zhongjing

Zhang Zhongjing (AD150 - 219) lived during the Eastern Han Dynasty. He resolved to become a physician after witnessing the ravages brought about by epidemics.

He was a high-ranking court official at some point. Even while he was posted to Changsha, he never neglected treating the people. At that time, court officials could not enter the residential area of the commoners at any time they wished to. And so Zhang Zhongjing would open the doors of the yamen on every first and 15th day of the lunar month so that he could provide consultation for the commoners. Patients from all over the land would travel to seek treatment from him.

Legend has it that dumplings, a traditional Chinese food, were invented by Zhang Zhongjing. Seeing how the poor suffered in the bitter cold and their ears became frostbitten, Zhang Zhongjing decided to wrap mutton, chilli and some warming medicinal herbs in dough skin.Folding them into the shape of an ear, he boiled them in water before giving them to the poor. Eating them warmed the body, promoted blood flow and thawed the cold ears. This medicine was called the 'Warming Ear Soup', and later dumplings.

Zhang Zhongjing later compiled experience culled from his practice and wrote 16 volumes of the *Treatise on Febrile and Miscellaneous Diseases*. It was China's earliest book to combine medical theories and medical experience, and provided analyses of the causes, symptoms, development and methods of handling acute febrile diseases in accordance with the theory of the Six Meridians.

More than 300 prescriptions and their effectiveness were recorded in the book. People called the prescriptions 'classic prescriptions'. His book also earned Zhang Zhongjing the title of 'Ancestor of Prescriptions' and the 'Ancestor of Medicine'. Practitioners of Chinese medicine still use his original prescriptions to treat diseases today.

* *Treatise on Febrile and Miscellaneous Diseases* has been lost through the ages. Wang Shuhe, a famous physician during the Jin Dynasty, rearranged the materials into two books — *Treatise on Febrile Diseases* and *Synopsis of Prescriptions of the Golden Chamber*.

> **Synopsis from Prescriptions of the Golden Chamber** — Decoction of Liquorice, Wheat and Jujube
>
> Ingredients: 10 g of liquorice, 30 g of wheat, 10 jujube
> Preparation: Cook them in 500 ml of water. Take it in three doses, one dose a day.
> Functions: Used as a sedative for neurosis, strengthens the spleen.
>
> The original decoction was to treat hysteria in women resulting from melancholy. It is now used to treat neurosis, schizophrenia, hysteria and menopause.

Zhang Zhongjing's Practice

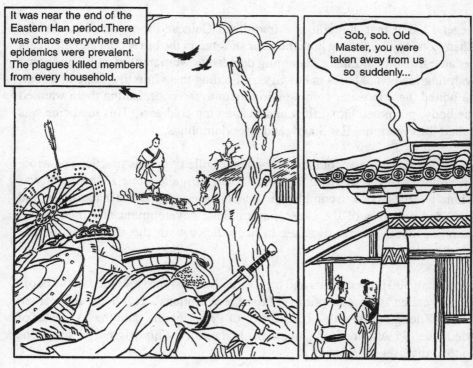

It was near the end of the Eastern Han period. There was chaos everywhere and epidemics were prevalent. The plagues killed members from every household.

Sob, sob. Old Master, you were taken away from us so suddenly...

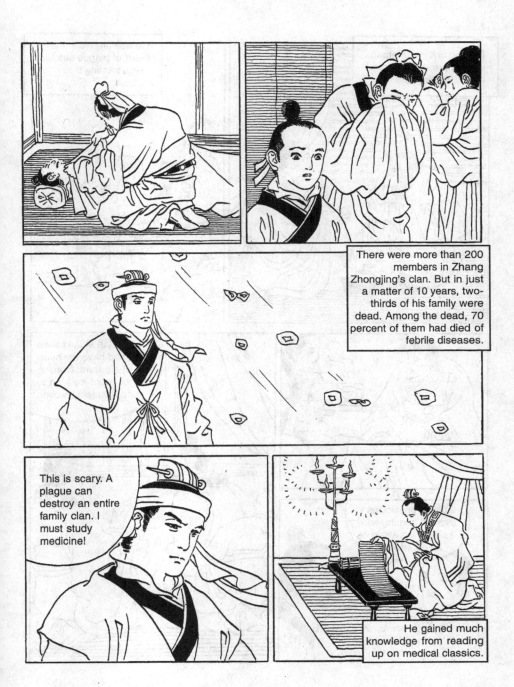

There were more than 200 members in Zhang Zhongjing's clan. But in just a matter of 10 years, two-thirds of his family were dead. Among the dead, 70 percent of them had died of febrile diseases.

This is scary. A plague can destroy an entire family clan. I must study medicine!

He gained much knowledge from reading up on medical classics.

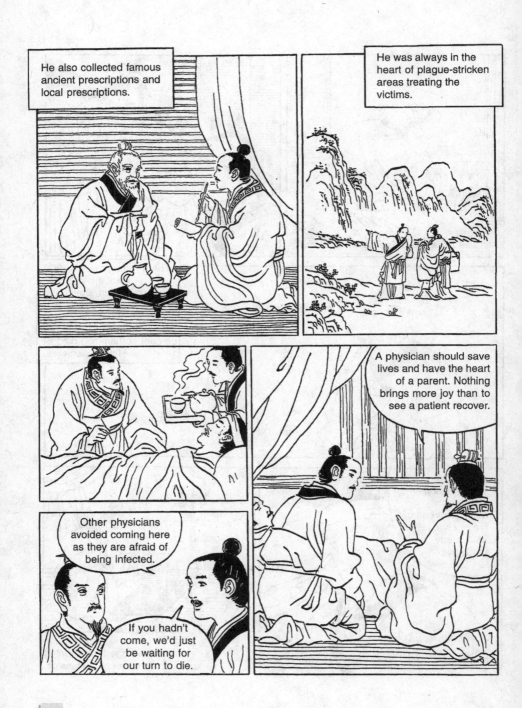

He also collected famous ancient prescriptions and local prescriptions.

He was always in the heart of plague-stricken areas treating the victims.

A physician should save lives and have the heart of a parent. Nothing brings more joy than to see a patient recover.

Other physicians avoided coming here as they are afraid of being infected.

If you hadn't come, we'd just be waiting for our turn to die.

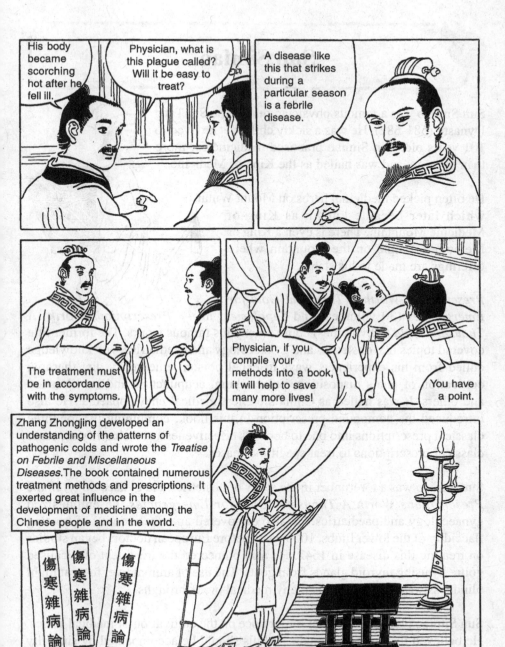

His body became scorching hot after he fell ill.

Physician, what is this plague called? Will it be easy to treat?

A disease like this that strikes during a particular season is a febrile disease.

The treatment must be in accordance with the symptoms.

Physician, if you compile your methods into a book, it will help to save many more lives!

You have a point.

Zhang Zhongjing developed an understanding of the patterns of pathogenic colds and wrote the *Treatise on Febrile and Miscellaneous Diseases*. The book contained numerous treatment methods and prescriptions. It exerted great influence in the development of medicine among the Chinese people and in the world.

傷寒雜病論
傷寒雜病論
傷寒雜病論

Sun Simiao

Sun Simiao was a famous physician during the Sui Tang Dynasty (581-682). He was a sickly child, yet he lived to 101 years old. Sun Simiao practised medicine for more than 80 years and was hailed as the King of Medicine.

He often picked medicinal herbs on Mount Wutai, which later became known as King of Medicine Mountain. There is even a King of Medicine Temple on the mountain where offerings are made to his statue.

Prescriptions Worth A Thousand Gold for Emergencies (30 volumes) and *Supplement to the Prescriptions Worth A Thousand Gold* (30 volumes) count among his famous works. The former title covered topics like obstetrics and gynaecology and paediatrics with knowledge culled from his experience, ways to expel poison, emergency diet therapy, cultivation of one's disposition, pulse taking, acupuncture and moxibustion and others. It was hailed as China's earliest medical encyclopaedia. He also introduced the compound prescription in this book, combining two or three classical prescriptions into one to boost its effectiveness, and simplifying some classical prescriptions to treat specific diseases.

Sun Simiao was a forerunner in the study of obstetrics and gynaecology. In the *Prescriptions Worth A Thousand Gold for Emergencies*, he emphasized gynaecology and paediatrics. He also discovered an effective way of treating flaccidity of the lower limbs, 1000 years before European doctors began studies on treating this disease in 1642. He also pioneered the treatment of localised goitre by using thyroid glands from goats. The use of animal liver to treat night blindness was also one of his many medical breakthroughs.

Sun Simiao placed paramount importance on the cultivation of medical ethics. He believed that excellent medical skills should be accompanied by sincerity of heart. His motto was: "Take decisive action tempered with careful thought, be flexible in according treatment, but never be subjective in one's judgement."

Sun Simiao:

"A life is worth a thousand taels of gold,
A life-saving prescription is worth more than a thousand taels of gold."

"Nothing is more precious than a person's life. It is worth more than a thousand gold. The merit a life-saving prescription earns is worth more than a thousand gold."

When he was a child, Sun Simiao suffered the ravages of illnesses and appreciated the importance of a physician. His famous works, *Prescriptions Worth A Thousand Gold for Emergencies* and *Supplement to the Prescriptions Worth A Thousand Gold* underline the value of life.

Sun Simiao — The Physician

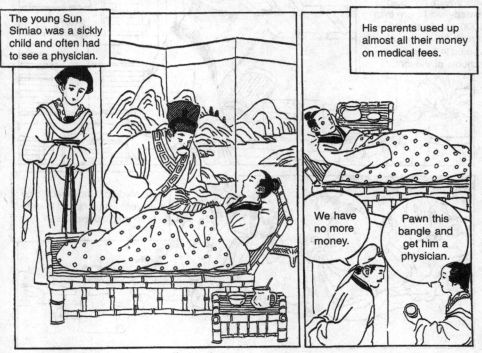

The young Sun Simiao was a sickly child and often had to see a physician.

His parents used up almost all their money on medical fees.

We have no more money.

Pawn this bangle and get him a physician.

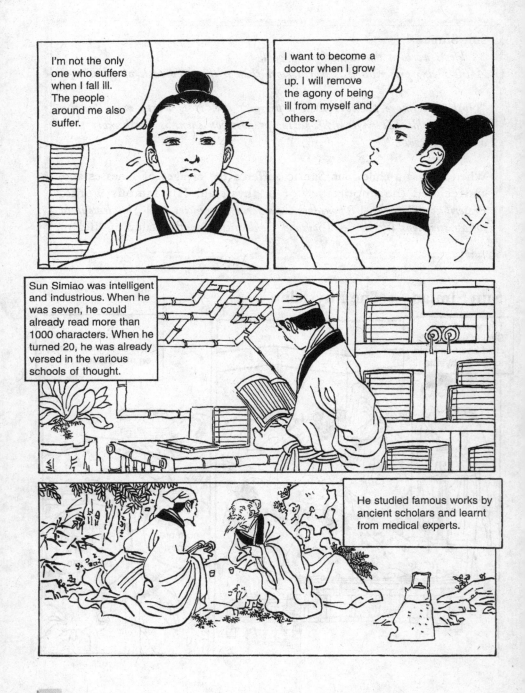

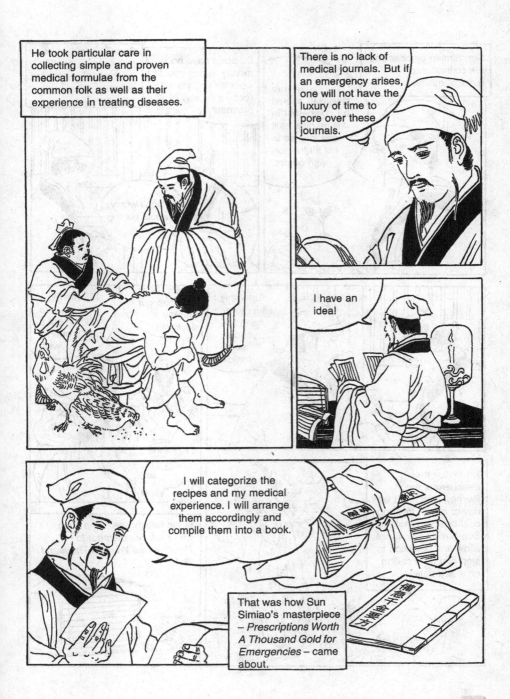

He took particular care in collecting simple and proven medical formulae from the common folk as well as their experience in treating diseases.

There is no lack of medical journals. But if an emergency arises, one will not have the luxury of time to pore over these journals.

I have an idea!

I will categorize the recipes and my medical experience. I will arrange them accordingly and compile them into a book.

That was how Sun Simiao's masterpiece – *Prescriptions Worth A Thousand Gold for Emergencies* – came about.

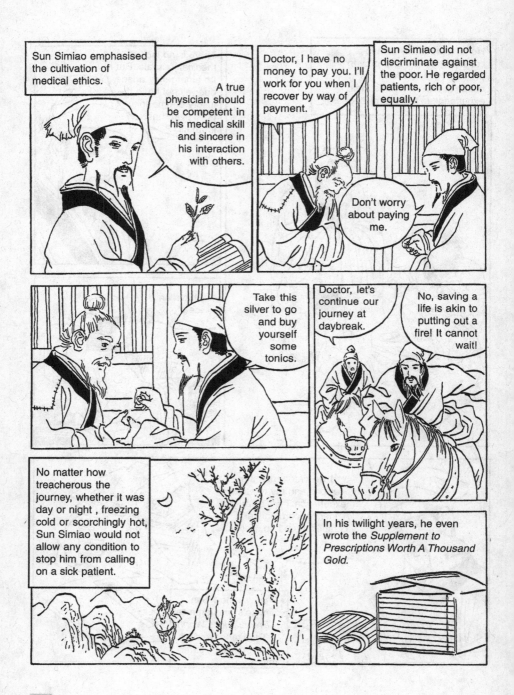

Zhu Danxi

Zhu Danxi was a famous physician who lived during the Yuan Dynasty (1281 - 1358). He was an excellent doctor and very often, one prescription from him would cure the patient. Hence the people called him 'Zhu One-Prescription' and 'Half-Immortal Zhu'.

Zhu Danxi only began to read up on medicine at 30 years of age as his mother suffered from a chronic pain in the spleen. Five years later, he cured his mother of her ailment.

When he was 36, he studied neo-Confucicanism under Xu Wenyi. In just a few years, he was known as an erudite Confucian scholar.

When Xu Wenyi fell gravely ill, he advised Zhu Danxi to switch to the study of medicine. Remembering how his own child, wife, younger brother, uncles and other family members had died at the hands of inept physicians, Zhu Danxi gave up his ambition to become a court official and switched to the study of medicine instead.

At that time, the *Prescriptions of the Drug Mixing Store* from the Song Dynasty given out by the authorities was all the rage. Inept physicians would just lift the medical formulae from the book blindly and prescribe them to patients. Zhu Danxi recognized the limitations of the book. So he studied *The Yellow Emperor's Medicine Classic*, *Difficult Classic* and others. He also travelled to other regions and called on renowned physicians. The renowned physician Luo Zhiti took him under his wing, and a few years later, Zhu Danxi had become a top physician with vast knowlege and consummate medical skills.

Zhu Danxi conceived the unique theory of nourishing the yin. It advocates nourishing the yin to lower the fire in one's body. He also opposed the indiscriminate use of pungent and warming medicines and stressed the importance of watching one's diet. His theories had widespread influence. Japanese medical experts specially visited China during the Ming Dynasty to learn from Danxi. Today, Japan still has societies founded on Danxi's teachings.

Zhu Danxi's Theory of Nourishing the Yin to Prepare for Old Age

Zhu Danxi believed that old age illness were due to insufficient yin and excess yang; hence he believed nourishing yin would expel fire and prevent sickness in old age.

"A person who has reached 60, 70 years of age will have depleted much of his vital essence and blood. Even if he is not suffering from poor diet or ill health, he is already suffering from the heat syndrome."

"Wufu pills should not be abused. Avoid wines and oily meat; grilled, smoked and fried food; spicy, sweet and oily food."

"The elderly have a deficiency of the spleen and insufficient yin. Heat in the stomach will cause hunger pangs; a weak spleen means poor food digestion and too much food will put stress on the stomach. Deficiency of yin will cause stagnation of the qi and result in diseases."

Zhu Danxi Studies Medicine

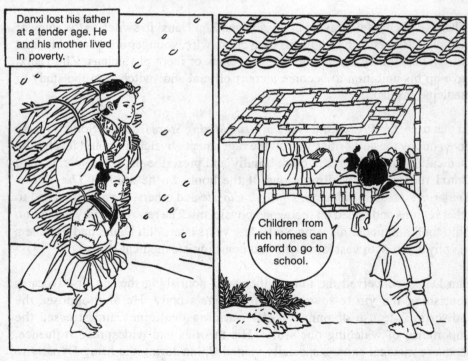

Danxi lost his father at a tender age. He and his mother lived in poverty.

Children from rich homes can afford to go to school.

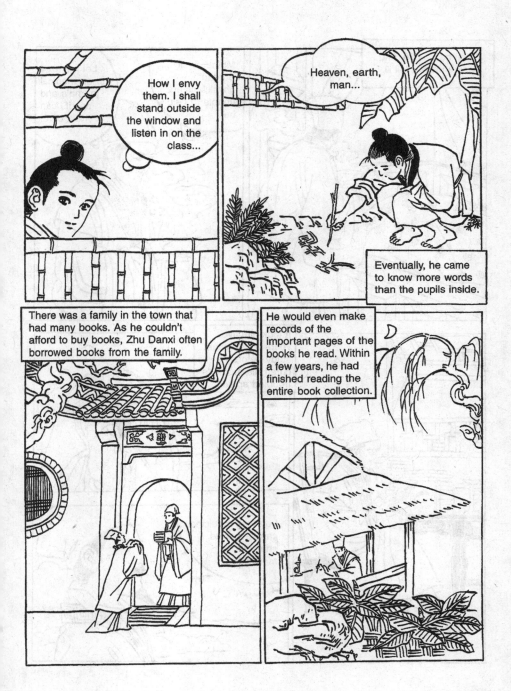

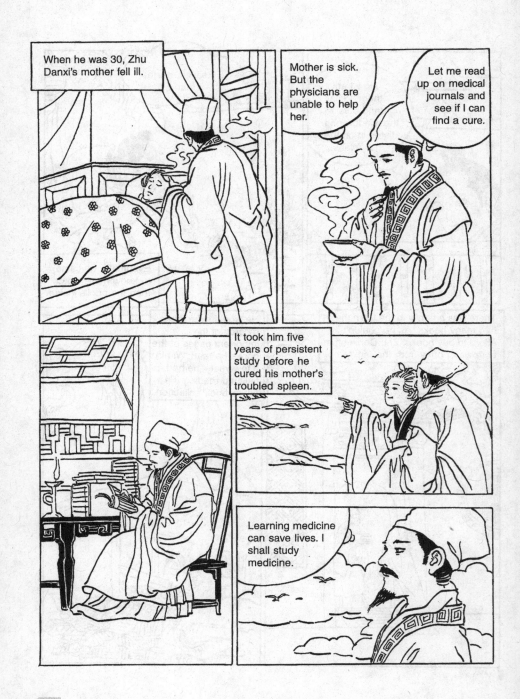

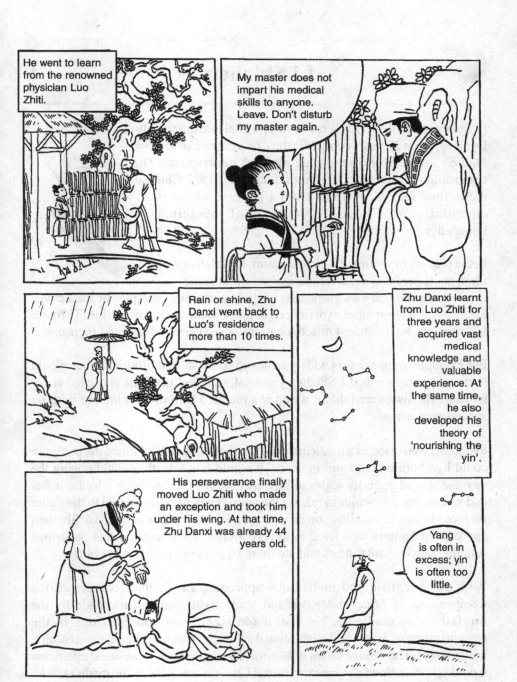

He went to learn from the renowned physician Luo Zhiti.

My master does not impart his medical skills to anyone. Leave. Don't disturb my master again.

Rain or shine, Zhu Danxi went back to Luo's residence more than 10 times.

Zhu Danxi learnt from Luo Zhiti for three years and acquired vast medical knowledge and valuable experience. At the same time, he also developed his theory of 'nourishing the yin'.

His perseverance finally moved Luo Zhiti who made an exception and took him under his wing. At that time, Zhu Danxi was already 44 years old.

Yang is often in excess; yin is often too little.

165

Li Shizhen

Li Shizhen (1518 - 1593), a renowned physician from the Ming Dynasty, spent 27 years compiling the *Compendium of Materia Medica* — the world-renowned medical masterpiece. The compendium comes in 52 volumes. It contains 1892 Chinese medicines and more than 1000 illustrations. It is a compilation of China's 2000 years of medicinal knowledge.

In the process of writing the compendium, Li Shizhen often made personal observations and travelled to the deep mountains and vast grasslands to study and collect samples of medicines. He also learnt from more experienced persons in the area of medicine. Through his research, he debunked misconceptions about certain drugs and their uses.

For example, *langmei* was widely believed to be an immortal fruit that would bestow eternal youth. Li Shizhen personally picked the fruit and tried it for himself. He discovered that it was just a mutated fruit of the elm tree with no special properties.

Pangolins were used as a medicinal drug. Earlier books had claimed the pangolin could live both on land and in water. It would feign death on land during the day and spread open its scales to lure ants into it, then go back into the water and spread open its scales to release the ants. When the ants floated to the water surface, it would swallow them as food. To verify this claim, Li Shizhen approached hunters who lived in the mountains. He found out that pangolins actually attacked ants' nests and ate them by sticking their tongue out.

With his scientific and meticulous approach, Li Shizhen completed the *Compendium of Materia Medica* and made right many errors made by the forefathers of medicine. He also made significant contributions in the categorisation of plants and other related sciences (biology, chemistry, geology, mineralogy). The *Compendium of Materia Medica* has been translated into many languages and helped advance traditional Chinese medicine in the medical field.

Medicinal diets in the *Compendium of Materia Medica*

Li Shizhen stressed medicinal diets to preserve health. Many medicinal food recipes were recorded in the *Compendium of Materia Medica*. Among the recipes was medicinal congee.

Walnut Congee
Ingredients: Walnut 60g, Millet 100g
Method: Crush the walnuts with the shells. Add some water and cook the millet into congee. Add the crushed walnut and cook until a film of oil forms on the surface of the congee. The congee should be taken warm twice a day.
Functions: It nourishes the kidneys and acts as an astringent for the lungs. It also moistens and replenishes the spleen and stomach.

Li Shizhen Compiles the *Compendium of Materia Medica*

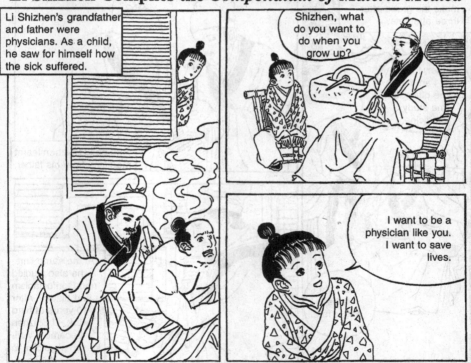

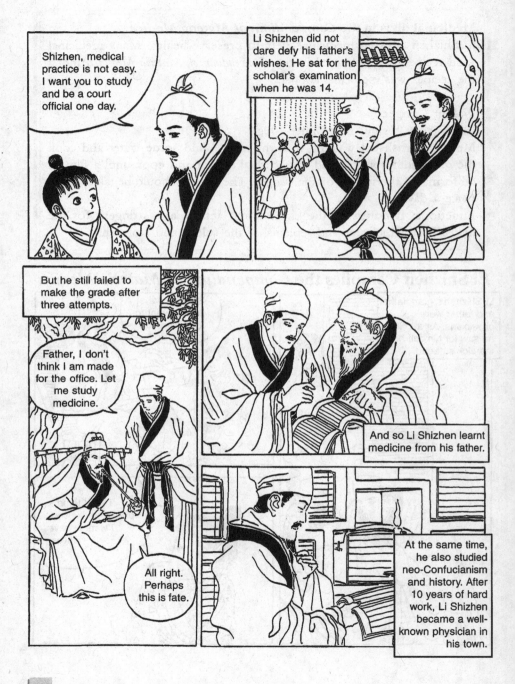

168

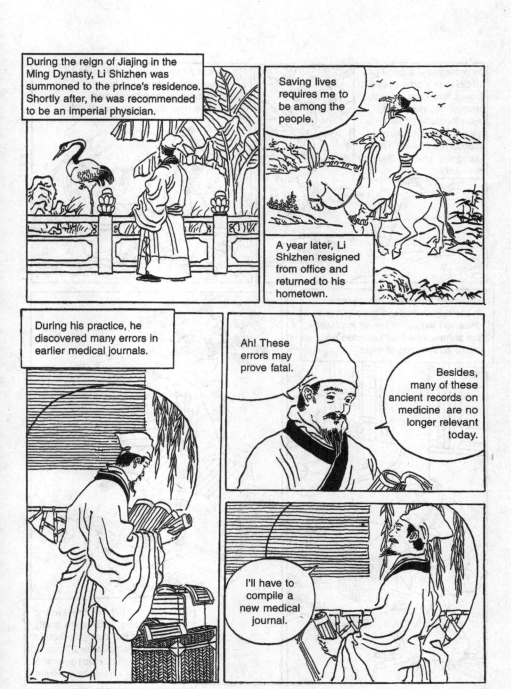

During the reign of Jiajing in the Ming Dynasty, Li Shizhen was summoned to the prince's residence. Shortly after, he was recommended to be an imperial physician.

Saving lives requires me to be among the people.

A year later, Li Shizhen resigned from office and returned to his hometown.

During his practice, he discovered many errors in earlier medical journals.

Ah! These errors may prove fatal.

Besides, many of these ancient records on medicine are no longer relevant today.

I'll have to compile a new medical journal.

In order to do a good job, Li Shizhen pored over 800 books including history, astronomy, medicine, astrology and others. He also travelled to many places like Henan, Hebei, Jiangnan, Hunan, Jiangsu and Anhui.

He consulted countless old farmers, fishermen, carpenters and hunters, collating medical knowledge and experience from the common folk.

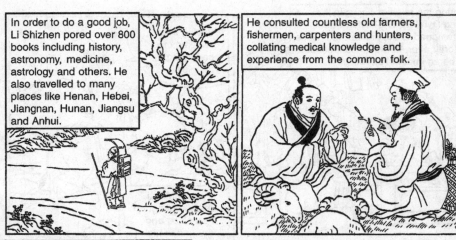

He would travel into the mountains in the day and spend the night in a deserted temple or house to classify the samples he had collected and make illustrations of them.

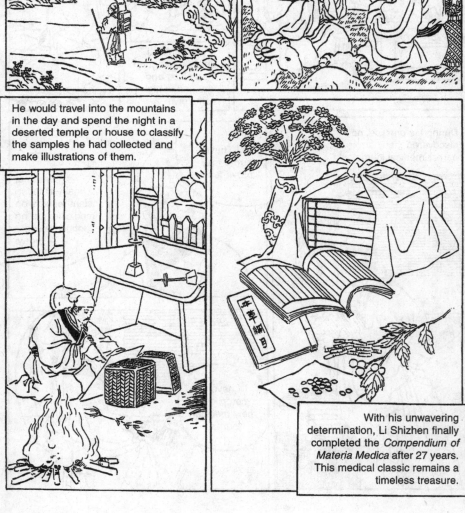

With his unwavering determination, Li Shizhen finally completed the *Compendium of Materia Medica* after 27 years. This medical classic remains a timeless treasure.

Ancient Female Physicians

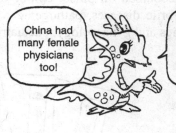

China had many female physicians too!

But very little was written about them. That is why few people know about them.

Chun Yuyan

This female physician of the Han Dynasty was an expert in obstetrics and gynaecology. It is said she helped the Empress of her time during childbirth.

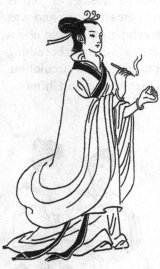

Bao Gu

A female physician during the Jin Dynasty. She was the wife of the famous academic Ge Hong. She learnt about medicine from her father and husband. She travelled widely to practise medicine and was especially good at moxibustion. The people later built a temple in her honour as a token of their gratitude towards her.

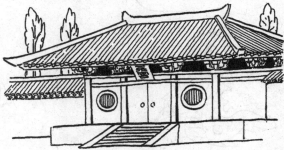

171

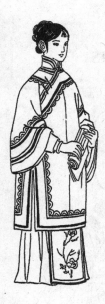

Zeng Yi

The Qing Dynasty female physician wrote the *Gu Huan Shi Volume* in three parts — *Book on Females*, *Book on Medicine* and *Book on Poetry and Prose*. The Book on Medicine discoursed on pulse, colour of tongue, acute infectious febrile diseases, pathogenic wind, pathogenic cold, obstetrics and gynaecology, paediatrics and surgery.

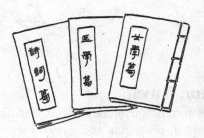

Zeng Yi was struck by epidemics four times. So she had a personal knowledge of pathogenic cold and symptoms of acute infectious febrile diseases as well as their respective treatments. She often made up her own prescriptions and was adept at it. Zeng Yi was also very particular about teaching the people about personal hygiene. She recommended rest to preserve mental strength, breathing fresh air to preserve the lungs and frequent exercise to promote blood circulation. Zeng Yi may be considered the greatest female physician in ancient China.

Chinese medicine is not a male-dominated field. Female doctors have also made contributions.

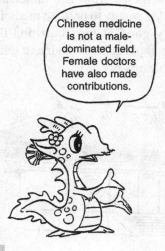

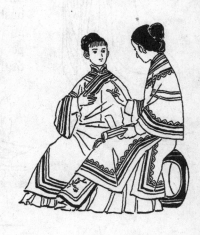

MODERNISATION OF CHINESE MEDICINE

The unique theories, diagnostic methods and treatment in traditional Chinese medicine contrast greatly with western medicine. In order to stay relevant in the modern-day context, besides preserving the best of its traditions, traditional Chinese medicine has gradually embarked on the road towards modernisation.

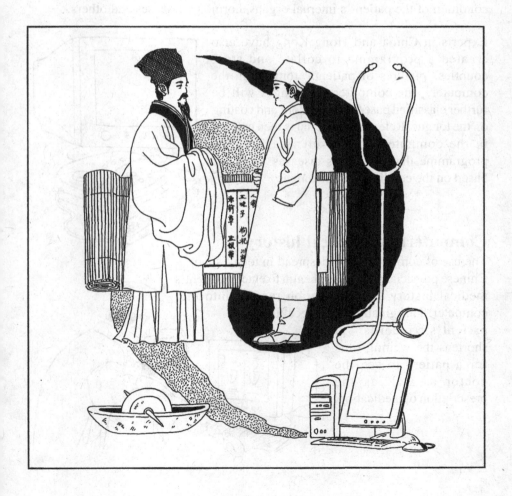

Diagnosis goes hi-tech

Besides employing the four traditional methods of diagnosis, modern traditional Chinese medicine has also started to adopt technological devices to aid in the diagnostic process. There are diagnostic devices for analysing the acupoints and research is being conducted on an automated system for pulse diagnosis.

The Electrodermal Screening Device (EDSD) is one of the electronic gadgets that was designed to read the systems of collaterals and meridians and acupoints in traditional Chinese medicine. The doctor measures the electrical resistance on an acupoint with a pen-like tool while the patient holds a hand electrode to complete the circuit with the EDSD. This way, he will be able to find out the condition of the patient's internal organs, hormonal releases and others.

Experts in China and Hong Kong have also created a programme to collate and store countless pictures of patients' tongues in the computer. The computerised images will be further classified based on the colour and coating on the tongue. Reference material is then entered in the computer. The result is a programme that diagnoses diseases based on the condition of the tongue.

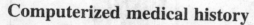

Computerized medical history

The use of computers is widespread in today's world. Chinese physicians have also begun to enter a patient's medical history and medication records into the computer. This greatly aids in recalling the patient's records and shortens the waiting time for a patient to see the doctor as well as the prescription of medication.

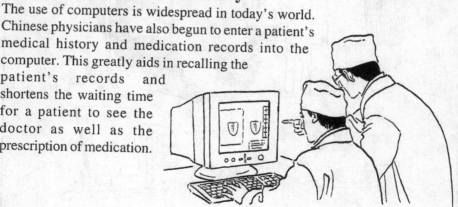

Chinese medicine in concentrate form

Chinese medicine often takes a long time to prepare. These days, Chinese medicine can be processed into a powder form with a strength from five to 15 times as concentrated. This not only ensures that the taste and efficacy of the medicine remains unaffected, it is also more economically viable.

Some medical halls also stock bottles of Chinese medicine concentrate. The pharmacist will dispense the concentrate based on the prescription given to him by the physician through the computer. The required quantity will then be packed in smaller bags and sealed before being dispensed to the patient.

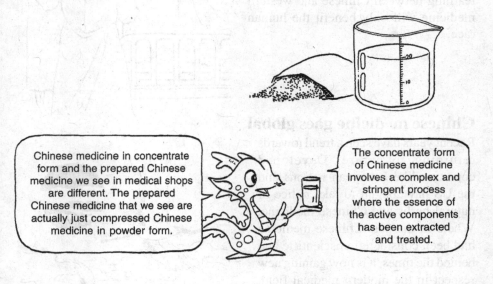

Chinese medicine in concentrate form and the prepared Chinese medicine we see in medical shops are different. The prepared Chinese medicine that we see are actually just compressed Chinese medicine in powder form.

The concentrate form of Chinese medicine involves a complex and stringent process where the essence of the active components has been extracted and treated.

Modern methods of decoction

To make things easier for the patients, some hospitals have installed special equipment to prepare Chinese medicine. High-pressure cookers will decoct the medicine before it is vacuum-sealed. Patients only have to reheat the medicine on reaching home before taking it. It is a fast and convenient ssytem and has done away with the time-consuming decoction of medicine.

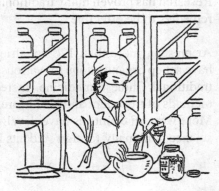

East meets West

Many integrated hospitals now offer both Chinese and western treatments to patients. They marry the two methods for greater efficacy in treating diseases. Some people have even called the modernisation of Chinese medicine and the marriage of Chinese and western medicine the Third Medical Science. This greater exchange of knowledge and learning between Chinese and western medicine will only benefit the human race.

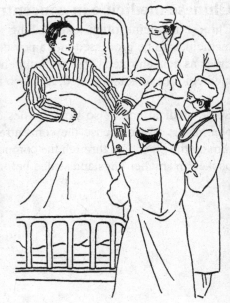

Chinese medicine goes global

Recent years have seen a trend towards returning to nature. Developed countries like European nations and the US have begun to take notice of natural herbs and Chinese medicine. Where in the past Chinese medicine had been considered unscientific and behind the times, it is now gaining new respect in the modern medical field. Research has proven many traditional remedies to be effective.

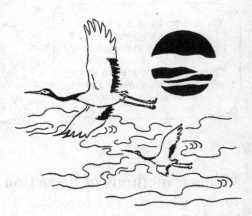

At present, more than 120 countries have set up organisations for various schools of alternative medicine, including traditional Chinese medicine. Increasingly, people are willing to accept the methods of treatment and healthcare practised in traditional Chinese medicine. More western countries have developed an interest in researching this ancient science, and many foreign students have gone to China to study it as well.

The Trademark of Chinese Medicine - The Yin-Yang Fish

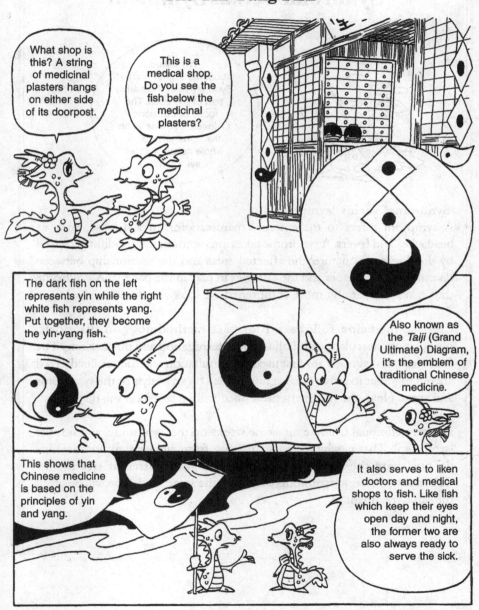

Syndrome versus Symptom

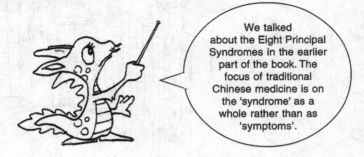

We talked about the Eight Principal Syndromes in the earlier part of the book. The focus of traditional Chinese medicine is on the 'syndrome' as a whole rather than as 'symptoms'.

'Syndrome' versus 'symptom'

A symptom refers to the external manifestation of a disease, such as headaches and fevers. A syndrome takes into account the conditions caused by the disease, its nature, the affected areas and the relationship between disease-causing factors and the energies in play in the patient. A syndrome thus takes a wider and more comprehensive look at a disease.

Chinese medicine follows a four-part methodology in diagnosis: observation, ausculation and olfaction, interrogation and pulse taking. The four steps of diagnosis are first used in consultation and the results derived are put together to arrive at a diagnosis based on an analyis of the symptoms and signs. Next, the treatment prescribed will be based on the diagnosis.

Hence, traditional Chinese medicine works on the 'syndrome' and not the 'symptom'. That is why patients suffering from similar symptoms which do not share the same syndrome will be given different treatments. Conversely, differing symptoms that share the same syndrome will be given the same treatment.

Appendix

The SARS outbreak

In Febuary 2003, reports began trickling in about an outbreak of a mysterious atypical pneumonia in China, which had already infected 300 people and claimed five lives. Soon, it was spreading through Asia, and in March, the World Health Organisation (WHO) issued a global alert on what was becoming known as Severe Acute Respiratory Syndrome (SARS).

The WHO began a global surveillance on cases of atypical pneumonia as cases continued to appear in other countries in Europe, Asia and the Americas. By the time the epidemic finally ended in July, the virus had claimed 916 lives out of a total number of 8422 infected persons*.

Traditional Chinese medicine and the fight against SARS

Though SARS is a new disease, traditional Chinese medicine has acquired much experience in fighting epidemics and diseases of a similar type through the ages, as evidenced by Zhang Zhongjing''s*Treatise on Febrile and Miscellaneous Diseases*, written well over 17 centuries ago.

In China, where the disease infected the greatest numbers, traditional Chinese medicine was combined with Western treatments to good effect. It was found to be most effective when started in the early stages of the disease, and in helping patients regain their strength during the recovery stage.

Here, in addition to acting directly to treat the disease, traditional Chinese medicine also helped to relieve pain, nausea and other side-effects of the Western treatments, especially as some of the Western medications used to suppress the virus also affected the body's own immune functions and cause the patient to become more susceptible to secondary infections from other pathogens.

* From the WHO summary: www.who.int/csr/sars/en/. Last updated 7 August 2003.

Defending against the threat of SARS

Though the SARS virus is in abeyance for now, some experts are concerned that the virus may return in the winter months, when the climate turns cooler again. Traditional Chinese medicine offers many preventive measures that can be taken to minimise your chances of succumbing to the disease.

In traditional Chinese medicine, SARS is classified as belonging to the heat syndrome with interior dampness, which act together to injure the qi in the lungs and bodily fluids quickly. Thus, treatment is centred on relieving internal heat, removing dampness, building qi and promoting the flow of fluids to detoxify the body.

Recipes to prevent SARS

Here are some tonic recipes to boost your immunity while reducing heat and dampness, taken from various websites on Chinese medicine.

Recipe 1	Recipe 2	Recipe 3
Honeysuckle 30g, woad root 10g, holly fern rhizome 10g, almond 10g, balloonflower root 10g, lilyturf root 15g, tangerine peel 6g, fresh liquorice 6g, chrysanthemum 6g.	Milkvetch root 10-12g, *baishu* 9g, ledebouriella root 6g, Japanese honeysuckle 9g, forsythia fruit 9g, reed rhizome 15-20g, mint 6g, platycodon root 6g, stir-baked liquorice 5g.	*Cangshu* 12g, *baishu* 15g, milkvetch root 15g, ledebouriella root 10g, giant hyssop 12g, glehnia root 15g, Japanese honeysuckle 20g, holly fern rhizome 12g.
Boil in 300ml of water for 15 minutes to condense it into 100ml. Take twice a day, morning and evening.	One dose a day, taken warm. Continue twice a day for five consecutive days.	Boil in water. Consume twice a day for seven to 10 consecutive days.
Recipe 4	**Recipe 5**	**Recipe 6**
Fresh reed rhizome 20g, Japanese honeysuckle 15g, forsythia fruit 15g, cicada slough 10g, white-stiff silkworm 10g, mint 6g, fresh liquorice 5g.	Rhizome of cyrtomium 10g, Japanese honeysuckle 10g, forsythia fruit 10g, woad leaf 10g, *suye* 10g, kudzu vine root 10g, giant hyssop 10g, *cangshu* 10g, eupatorium 10g, pseudostarwort root 15g.	Honeysuckle 15g, forsythia fruit 15g, schizonepeta 15g, woad root 15g, houttuynia 30g, ledebouriella root 12g, mint 12g, skullcap root 12g, wild chrysanthemum 15g, liquorice 6g.
Boil in water and drink as a tea. Continue for seven to 10 consecutive days.	Boil in water and take twice a day for seven to 10 consecutive days.	Soak for 30 minutes and bring to boil over a slow fire (add mint 10 minutes later) for 15 minutes. Take in three doses over three days.

Acupressure and moxibustion

The *zusanli* acupoint, which can be found in both legs, strengthens the spleen and removes dampness.

Moxibustion

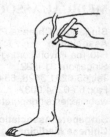

- Light the moxa and place the moxa stick on the *zusanli* acupoints on both legs for five to 10 minutes.
- Do it one or two times a day for five consecutive days.

How to find it:

The *zusanli* acupoint is on the outer leg, three inches below the knee-cap. It is about one finger breath away from the front of the shin-bone.

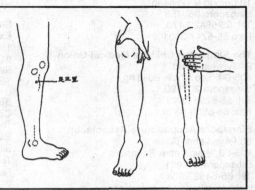

Acupresssure

Use both thumbs to press on the *zusanli* acupoint. Repeat the action 108 times until you feel soreness on that spot.

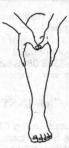

Caution

Before taking any medicine, it is best to consult a physician first to make sure it suits your constitution. Remember, do not consume more than what is necessary! Also, moxibustion should only be carried out by professionals.

CHINESE MEDICINE RESOURCES DIRECTORY

MEDICAL ASSOCIATIONS

Singapore Chinese Physicians' Association
640 Toa Payoh Lorong 4
Singapore 319522
Tel: 65-6251 3428, 65-6251 3304
Fax: 65-6254 0037
website: en.singaporetcm.com

Singapore Association for Promoting Chinese Medicine
10 Lorong 9 Geylang
Singapore 388758
Tel: 65-6842 5470
Fax: 65-6741 3301

The Singapore Chinese Medical Union
21 Tyrwhitt Road
#05-04, Foo Chow Building
Singapore 207530
Tel: 65-6296 2645
Fax: 65-6536 5520

Singapore Acupuncture Association
60 Paya Lebar Road
#05-08, Paya Lebar Square
Singapore 409051
Tel: 65-6452 2988
website: www.acupuncture.org.sg

Society of Traditional Chinese Medicine (Singapore)
BIK 333 Kreta Ayer Road #01-12/13
Singapore 080333
Tel: 65-6323 0898/6225 2246
website: www.society-tcms.org

The Medicine Manufacturer Association of Singapore
132 Neil Road
Singapore 088861
Tel: 65-6224 5379
website: medmfg.org.sg

Singapore Chinese Druggists Association
119 Tyrwhitt Road
Singapore 207547
Tel: 65-6298 4740
Fax: 65-6299 3528
website: scda.org.sg

Singapore Chinese Drug Importers & Exporters Guild
151 Chin Swee Road
#15-02, Manhattan House
Singapore 169876
Tel: 65-6735 2983

Singapore Chinese Physicians' Training College Alumnus Association
Toa Payoh Central
P.O. Box 134
Singapore 913105
Tel: 65-6569 3905
Fax: 65-6256 3608

Singapore Chinese Medicines and Health Products Merchant Association
346A King George's Avenue
Singapore 208577
Tel: 65-6293 8019
Fax: 65-6293 5803
website: www.tcm.org.sg

MEDICAL INSTITUTES AND PRACTITIONERS

Singapore Thong Chai Medical Institution
50 Chin Swee Road
Thong Chai Building #01-01
Singapore 169874
Tel: 65-6733 6905
Fax: 65-6733 3552
website: www.stcmi.org.sg

Traditional Chinese Medicine Practitioners Board
website: www.healthprofessionals.gov.sg/content/hprof/tcmpb/en.html

Singapore Chung Hwa Medical Institution
No. 640 Toa Payoh Lorong 4
Singapore 319522
Tel: 65-6251 3304
Fax: 6254 0037
website: www.chunghwamedicalinstitution.com

CHINESE MEDICINE COURSES

Singapore College of Traditional Chinese Medicine
640 Toa Payoh Lor 4
Singapore 319522
Tel: 65-6250 3088
Fax: 6356 9901
website: www.singaporetcm.edu.sg
Professional courses in Chinese medicine.

TCM College (Singapore) Pte Ltd
371 Beach Road #02-37 Keypoint
Singapore 199597
Tel: 65-6227 9969
Fax: 65-6299 3294
Training school for Chinese Medicinal Materials Dispensers.

This listing is intended to be a resource for anyone with an interest in traditional Chinese medicine. If you wish to have your organisation or company included, please submit the name, address and contact information for your organization in English and Chinese. Listing is free. Thank you!

Fax: **6392 6455**
Email: **asiapacbooks@pacific.net.sg**

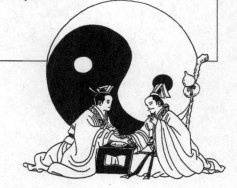

WEB RESOURCES

Greater China Herbs
www.greaterchinaherbs.com
In English, Chinese, Japanese and Korean. It offers diet therapy, medicinal diets, tips on healthcare etc.

Traditional Chinese Medicine Basics
http://www.tcmbasics.com/
Learning resource for traditional Chinese medicine, with introductions to many fundamental theories.

Comprehensive Services of Traditional Chinese Medicine
http://www.tcmtreatment.com/
Online sale of books and herbs, with explanations and treatment advice for common aliments and an introduction to commonly used herbs.

Qi: The Journal of Traditional Eastern Health and Fitness
http://qi-journal.com/
Information on traditional Chinese medicine, including acupuncture, *qigong*, herbs, *taijiquan*. Also contains sections on Chinese culture and philosophy.

Printed in the United States
By Bookmasters